The Gene and the Genie

Carolina Academic Press
Medical Anthropology Series

Pamela J. Stewart *and* Andrew Strathern
Series Editors

Curing and Healing
Medical Anthropology in Global Perspective
Andrew Strathern *and* Pamela Stewart

Physicians at Work, Patients in Pain, 2nd Edition
Biomedical Practice and Patient Response in Mexico
Kaja Finkler

Healing the Modern in a Central Javanese City
Steve Ferzacca

Elusive Fragments
Making Power, Propriety and Health in Samoa
Douglass D. Drozdow-St. Christian

Endangered Species
Health, Illness, and Death Among Madagascar's People of the Forest
Janice Harper

The Practice of Concern
Ritual, Well-Being, and Aging in Rural Japan
John W. Traphagan

The Gene and the Genie
Tradition, Medicalization and Genetic Counseling
in a Bedouin Community in Israel
Aviad E. Raz

Social Discord and Bodily Disorders
Healing Among the Yupno of Papua New Guinea
Verena Keck

The Gene and the Genie

Tradition, Medicalization and Genetic Counseling in a Bedouin Community in Israel

Aviad E. Raz
BEN-GURION UNIVERSITY OF THE NEGEV

CAROLINA ACADEMIC PRESS
Durham, North Carolina

Library of Congress Cataloging-in-Publication Data

Raz, Aviad E., 1968-
The gene and the genie : tradition, medicalization, and genetic counseling in a Bedouin community in Israel / by Aviad E. Raz.
p. cm.
Includes bibliographical references.
ISBN 0-89089-448-5
1. Genetic counseling -- Israel. 2. Bedouins -- Medical care -- Israel. I. Title.

RB155.7.R39 2004
362.196'042'095694--dc22

2003027142

Carolina Academic Press
700 Kent Street
Durham, North Carolina 27701
Telephone (919) 489-7486
Fax (919) 493-5668
www.cap-press.com

Printed in the United States of America
Cover Design by Erin M. Ehman

Contents

List of Tables and Figures

Tables

Figures

Medical Anthropology Series Editors' Preface

Pamela J. Stewart and Andrew Strathern

In Aviad Raz's book we see an issue of global concern, i.e., genetic counseling, being analyzed in relation to religion, ethics, morality, and medical practice. The practices of genetic counseling, in terms of biomedicine, are themselves continuously changing as new developments in human genetics (e.g., new technologies and further research in mapping the human genome) occur. Numbers of different genetic screening tests are available to patients, including prenatal tests that screen for disorders in the fetus, carrier testing to check for the possibility of an individual carrying a particular genetic marker, and susceptibility tests to determine if a person is at higher risk of developing a particular disease. The philosophy of genetic counseling is impacted by a myriad of complex ethical, social, legal, religious, and educational issues. The specific location of the project presented in this book is a Bedouin Community in Israel but the implications and considerations are ones that apply to many other areas, e.g., the USA, Canada, Europe, the Pacific, etc.

Genetic counseling is a growing field in which health care professionals, working in conjunction with a team of health care workers, offer information and provide support to families who have members with birth defects or genetic disorders, or to individuals who are affected with a genetic condition, or to families in high risk categories for genetically transmitted health conditions. The type of advice offered to patients varies but may include: ways to comprehend medical diagnosis; information on the mechanisms by which heredity contributes to a disorder and the risk of a recurrence in particular relatives; explanations of alternatives available to patients for dealing with risk of recurrence; suggestions of particular courses of action which take into consideration the moral and religious feelings of the patients and their family; and means by which the affected person(s) can make life adjustments to the disorder or the possible risk of recurrence of a disorder.

One of the dilemmas involved in genetic testing and counseling is the question of how genetic information alters an individual's sense of "self" in terms of their relationship to others and their religious beliefs about wellness and morality. Other concerns are how genetic information may be used to a patient's disadvantage through genetic discrimination in regard to health insurance or employment, eligibility to marry and procreate, or loss of medical history privacy in general.

Aviad Raz's ethnographic explorations of the considerations and concerns over genetic testing and counseling in his research community are deftly presented. This work will be of interest to the general reader, those interested in health care practices, and also as a text to supplement courses on bioethics, applied medical anthropology, critical medical anthropology, and genetic ethics.

Of particular interest in this study is Raz's discussion of the role played by Bedouin marriage practices, specifically the norm of patrilateral cousin marriage, along with a religiously based ban on abortion. He portrays the processes whereby both counselors and marriage partners negotiate and exercise agency over their problems in relation to these roles. Similar problems are faced by parents in places such as Saudi Arabia where spinal muscular atrophy can result from consanguineous marriage patterns. "Consanguinity" in Raz's usage, usually refers to these patterns.

We are very pleased to include Aviad Raz's book in the Ethnographic Studies in Medical Anthropology Series. The other titles in this Series include:

"Curing and Healing: Medical Anthropology in Global Perspective", 1999 (by Andrew Strathern and Pamela J. Stewart).

"Healing the Modern in a Central Javanese City", 2001 (by Steve Ferzacca)

"Physicians at Work, Patients in Pain, 2nd edition", 2001 (by Kaja Finkler).

"Endangered Species: Health, Illness and Death among Madagascar's People of the Forest", 2002 (by Janice Harper).

"Elusive Fragments: Making Power, Propriety, and Health in Samoa", 2002 (by Douglass Drozdow-St. Christian).

"The Practice of Concern: Ritual, Well-Being, and Aging in Rural Japan," 2004 (by John W. Traphagan).

"Social Discord and Bodily Disorders: Healing Among the Yupno of Papua New Guinea," 2005 (by Verena Keck).

May 2003
Department of Anthropology
University of Pittsburgh
Pittsburgh, PA 15260
USA

Acknowledgments

The two worlds studied in this book comprise people whose help and cooperation have kept this research going. I am grateful to the many members of the Bedouin community studied here, who devoted precious time to my inquiries and were kind enough to let me into their homes and their lives. This study would not have been possible without their help and hospitality. I am particularly grateful to 'Abd al-Muaati al-Sāyyed and Dina Shahāda, whose contribution as community-outreach assistants was invaluable. I am equally indebted to the health professionals who introduced me to the genetics project and shared their thoughts and quandaries with me. I am indebted to Ha'lil al-Ba'dūr, Ā'māl abu-Sā'ad, Hana Beit-Or, and all the genetic counselors at the Genetics Institute. I would like to acknowledge the cooperation of Rivka Carmi and Ilana Shoham-Vardi, who initiated and oversaw the project described here and who were responsible for the tremendous genetic and epidemiological work that preceded this project. This study could not have taken place without their collaboration, and it benefited from their wisdom and experience. Thanks to Joel Zlotogora for explaining his approach to community genetics and the uses of the "Family Tree" software program in data analysis.

I am grateful to Marcela Ātar, Maya Rodnāi, and Muhammad al-Dāda, my graduate students at the Dept. of Behavioral Sciences, Ben-Gurion University, for their help in data collection and analysis. Special thanks go to Marcela, whose research skills and insights helped to shape the ideas and analyses that appear here. This research contains data collected by Marcela as part of her PhD study, a study she is presently pursuing in order to further explore the issue of genetic counseling to the Bedouin.

Among my academic colleagues, I am particularly indebted to Gideon Kressel, who saw the potential in this study and sharpened my perception of the culture of cousin marriage. The International Workshop on Health and Illness in Middle-East Societies, organized in April–May 2002 by A'ref Abu-Rabi'a in the Dept. of Middle-East Studies at Ben-Gurion University of the Negev, provided a well-appreciated opportunity for sharing my ideas. I am also grateful to Ruth Chadwick for her useful comments on earlier versions.

My bioethical sensibilities were shaped in discussions held at the Advanced European Bioethics Course "Ethics and Genetics," November 2000, at the University of Nijmegen, The Netherlands. I am particularly grateful, in this context, to Roberto Del'Orro, Nora Groce and Eric Juengst, who strengthened my conviction that bioethics should be studied in the community. Thanks are due, as always, to Norman Denzin for planting the seed of symbolic interactionism in me and for cultivating it through his continuing support. I am indebted to Pamela Stewart and Andrew Strathern, co-editors of this Medical Anthropology Series, for their close reading of the manuscript and incisive comments. This study was funded by grants from the Israel Foundation Trustees (project PS14/3) and the Israel Science Foundation (grant # 769/00-2) for which, needless to say, I am very grateful.

As always, I am deeply grateful to my wife, Ayala, for her continuing support, and to my sons, Orr, Yoav and Hillel, for the strength and happiness they give me.

Large portions of the following papers are reprinted in this book by permission of the publisher. Raz, Aviad & Marcela Atar, (2004), "Upright Generations of the Future," Journal of Contemporary Ethnography 33(3): 296–323, Sage Publications, Inc.; Raz, Aviad (2003), "Āysha: Genetics Education and Community Engagement in a Consanguineous Arab-Bedouin Population in Israel," Health: The Inter-Disciplinary Journal for the Social Study of Health and Illness 7(4): 32–56, Sage Publications Ltd; Raz, Aviad & Marcela Atar, (2003), "Nondirectiveness and Its Lay Interpretations: The Effect of Counseling Style, Ethnicity and Culture on Attitudes towards Genetic Counseling," Journal of Genetic Counseling, 12(4): 313–31, Kluwer Academic/ Plenum Publishers; and Raz, Aviad, Atar, Marcela, Rodnai, Maya, Shoham-Vardi, Ilana & Rivka Carmi, (2003), "Between Acculturation and Ambivalence: Knowledge of and Attitudes towards Genetic Counseling in an Arab-Bedouin Population in Israel," Community Genetics 193, S. Karger AG, Basel.

A.E.R

Introduction

The development of genetics is exerting a tremendous impact on our society, health, and culture. While this impact is expected to increase, we are still largely ignorant of its social, legal and ethical implications. James Watson, co-discoverer of the double helix structure of DNA and founding father of the Human Genome Project, was cited as saying: "We used to think our fate was in the stars. We now know, in large part, it is in our genes" (Conrad and Gabe, 1999: 1). In this study I examine what happens when this newly discovered scientific notion of "fate" encounters its traditional and religious conception. Can the traditional and the modern mix in any way, or are they doomed to fight for domination? The word "gene," which has no equivalent in Arabic and was therefore used as such in genetic instruction to the Bedouin community studied here, sounds like the Arabic word "*jinn.*" This coincidence had intriguing consequences, since *jinn* in Arabic folklore are spiritual beings that can take the form of either a demon or a genie.[1] Some of the Arabic-speaking counselors actually used this homophony for the purposes of instruction, telling their Bedouin audience that the gene is indeed something invisible and hidden that has great influence over the person's destiny.

The "gene/*jinn*" is a two-faced symbolic facade. I use it in the title to capture the paradoxical, yet very real, mixture of Bedouin tradition ("the *jinn*") and biomedicine ("the gene"). This exotic match can be read as reproducing the essential difference between East and West, local Bedouin culture and global biomedical culture. My intention is quite the opposite. As the ensuing study sets out to show, the "*jinn*" and the "gene" are discursive themes within

1. *Jinni*, feminine *jinniyah*, plural *jinn*, in Arabic and Islamic folklore, spirit or demon endowed with supernatural power. In ancient belief the *jinn* were associated with the destructive forces of nature. In Islamic tradition they were corporeal spirits similar to men in appearance but having certain supernatural powers, especially those of changing in size and shape. Capable of both good and evil, the *jinn* were popular in literatures of the Middle East, notably in the stories of the Thousand and One Nights. The term genie is the English form and is sometimes confused with the Roman *genius*.

a negotiated order. Rather than remaining different and detached, they are subjected to mutual modification and hybridization. Far from being pre-determined, their meaning is continuously reconstructed within micro-political circumstances and personal agendas.

The juxtaposition of the *jinn*/gene entails additional oppositions such as culture and nature as well as religion (spiritualism, fate) and science (mechanization, determinism). The "genie in the gene" could be seen in that respect as alluding to "the ghost in the machine." In the modern, biomedical perspective that seeks local compliance, the "genie in the gene" (namely genetic counseling) is to be conceived of as a *Deus ex machina*. Yet despite the counselor's role as information provider, instructor and guide, genetic counseling could also be perceived as eugenic and coercive. At a time when mapping the human genome is considered by many as an epitome of scientific progress, we also need a moral map of the debates in the domain of genetic counseling and public health. Genetic counseling, especially when targeting at-risk non-western populations, raises questions that are fundamental to bioethics, such as: What are the moral criteria for mandating genetic screening? Who decides when the disease is 'severe' enough? Can local values and/or perceptions of beneficence justify compromising nondirectiveness? And is eugenics always morally unacceptable?

There is a growing discussion of the impact of genetics on public health policies (e.g., Khoury et al., 2000; WHO, 2002). Sociologists have studied genetic counseling as a profession with a focus on the bioethical dilemmas of counselor-client interaction, especially in regard to selective abortion and the so-called 'tentative pregnancy' (Rothman 1986; Boss, 1993; Sutton, 1990; Bosk, 1992). There have been many sociological and cultural studies of the public images and discourses around the 'new genetics,' and the lay-professional disjunction of understanding (Conrad & Gabe, 1999; Nelkin and Lindee, 1995; Van Dijck, 1998). However, there is still no full-fledged ethnographic study of the development, implementation and reception of a community-based genetic counseling program.

Despite its espoused ideology of nondirectiveness and patient's autonomy, the intention of genetic counseling, on both the community and the individual level, is eugenicist by implication. There is an ethical paradox inherent in the practice of genetic counseling. Governmental pressures to lower health-care costs remain a stimulus to eugenic approaches, which are built into genetic counseling because of the normativity of medicine. Analysis of actual counseling sessions indicates that nondirectiveness is seldom accomplished and that the mechanism of informed consent does not work in reality. There is a need to develop a new paradigm for the ethical and social principles of genetic counseling, not only for individuals but also for the participation of communities.

This study concerns itself with "community genetics." While genetic counseling has been created for individual purposes, in reality it also involves the spouse, the family, and the community. However, scholars have seldom started with a conceptualization of the role of community and then focused on its interplay with individual concepts such as autonomy and consent. Genetic communities are a global phenomenon that juxtaposes a common genetic pool, ethnic bonds and political circumstances, e.g., African Americans, Native Americans, Asian immigrants, communities of "guest workers" (e.g., people from Turkey who live and work in Germany), the Amish, Ashkenazi Jews, Scottish clans, island communities, the Bedouin, and so on. Genetic communities can also be formed through voluntary associations and around support foundations. While genetic research takes special importance in consanguineous communities where endogamy increases the prevalence of recessive genetic diseases, such communities often have traditional values that are incongruent with the "standard view" of genetic counseling. In many such communities, consent cannot simply be "informed" but depend on instruction, individuals are often not "autonomous" but depend on others (especially the father), prearranged consanguineous marriages are a traditional norm, and abortion is often banned by religion. On the other hand, certain norms may constitute a "red line" that should not be morally or politically supported, such as the commercial use of prenatal or pre-implantation diagnosis for sex selection.

The ethical dilemmas of genetic counseling can be further framed within the communitarian-liberal debate. Different people behind the recent communitarian renaissance in the US have argued that moral life is rooted in the norms of particular communities. Liberalism, in contrast, has sought for norms that are universal and generalizable (similar to the conception of the "standard view" in genetic counseling). While liberals argue that communitarianism is likely to be parochial and sectarian, communitarians claim that liberalism is a "view from nowhere" that is more likely to produce rootlessness and anomie than justice. Without subscribing to either approach, I am interested in studying the impact of communal ends on the reasoning of individuals in genetic counseling issues. Locating the ethical, social and policy dimensions of genetic counseling within the communitarian/liberal debate is a project that has not yet been done.

This book offers an ethnography of genetic counseling in a traditional, inbred population of Negev Bedouin in Israel. The Negev Bedouin are a Moslem-Arab minority (estimated population around 130 000) residing in the southern part of Israel. Since the 1950s and increasingly after 1967 the Bedouin have been undergoing a rapid process of transition from a semi-nomadic to a sedentary, westernized way of life. In 2000 about 50% of the population lived in seven towns—Rahat, Tel al-Saba (Tel-Sheva), Kuseifa, 'Ar'ara, Shqeb al-Salam (Segev Shalom), Hura, and Laqiya—which were planned for them by Israeli governments, while the rest lived in scattered encampments and shantytowns. These formally "unrecognized" villages were created as a result of the refusal of the Bedouin to leave the land where they have been living for many years. Since the Israeli government does not officially recognize them as villages, they are denied basic services such as water, electricity, and sewage, and only a few have schools and clinics. Over 35 inherited diseases, with about 10 more familial mental retardation disorders of unknown etiology have so far been identified in the Bedouin community (Carmi et all, 1998). Infant mortality among the Bedouin is about 13.1 per 1000 live births (about 3.5 times more than the Jewish population), with about 50% due to congenital defects and hereditary diseases (Weitzman et al., 2000).

The Bedouin community is characterized by two important norms that directly affect genetic counseling: (a) preferred patrilateral parallel cousin marriage, which is the main reason for a high prevalence of genetic diseases; and (b) a religious ban on abortion. The counseling program offered to the Bedouin followed the scheme of "*Dor Yeshorim*" (literally, upright generations in Hebrew), a successful program that was developed in the orthodox-Ashkenazi Jewish community. Both programs consist of premarital screening and confidential storage of the results in a system that is used for carrier matching. Potential partners are told if they are genetically "compatible" or not ("incompatibility" meaning the two partners are carriers), without disclosing individual carrier status. In other words, such premarital carrier matching is a form of genetic counseling in which two individuals are told, if both are carriers, that they have a 25% risk at each pregnancy of having a child affected by the disease for which they were tested. If only one individual is a carrier this information is not disclosed. Carrier testing and matching were offered to the Bedouin mainly for two prevalent conditions: congenital hearing loss and beta-thalassemia (a genetically determined disorder characterized by reduced production of beta-globin chains, thus usually causing severe anemia). In the case of thalassemia, attempts for community engagement have only begun during the research period. There are many other genetic tests offered to the larger Bedouin population by the Genetic Institute at the local hospital, most of which are not part of the program for carrier matching, which was an experimental research project rather than a policy decision. An ongoing genetic research project attempts to discover a test for other inherited diseases prevalent in the targeted Bedouin sub-population, which could then be added to the existing experimental programs for carrier matching. Congenital hearing loss and thalassemia represent different paradigms in terms of the disease, its severity and social construction, and the cultural aspects of at-risk communities where the disease is prevalent. While focusing on the more established (and debated) counseling program for congenital hearing loss, I will use the thalassemia program for comparison.

This study provides a unique opportunity to examine, *in situ*, the interplay between medical science and tradition, medicalization and resistance, paternalism and empowerment, ethnic ties and bureaucratic rationality. While all counselors principally subscribed to the "standard view" of genetic counseling, in practice their attitudes ranged from an acceptance of directiveness (justified through a communitarian/utilitarian ethics) to an emphasis on the patient's autonomy. The attitudes of community members were broadly divided into utilization, compliance, and rejection. These grounded categories will be analyzed on the basis of in-depth interviews conducted with counselors and community members, as well as observations of counseling and instruction sessions. The book will show how the community has selectively adopted genetic counseling according to its own agendas and within the broader context of its culture. The narratives of rejection, compliance and utilization reveal conflicts and tensions between the rationality of biomedical interventions and the wider heterogeneous social framework to which people respond in their decision-making processes.

Using a combination of qualitative and quantitative methods, this study sets out to analyze the social organization of communal and medical discourses, highlighting differences between public attitudes and backstage decisions. Such an analysis can offer a more fine-tuned identification of patterns and predictors of participation in all stages of genetic testing and counseling by various segments of the population. The approach also has wider implications. Understanding the cultural factors and discourses through which the community comes to terms with genetic testing and counseling can contribute to our ability to use and implement genetic research in public health programs for ethnic enclaves and traditional societies worldwide, and particularly in the Middle East.

While the program studied here takes place in a part of the world that is relatively distant and unfamiliar to most readers, its implications are not so remote. Although my focus in this study is particular, I believe that the moral is general. I share Tan Alora and Lumitao's (2001: 3) contention that "the bioethics that developed in the US in the 1970s and 1980s and purports to provide a global bioethics that is applicable in all countries falls seriously short of this goal." Screening programs are becoming a normative part of life in third, second and first world settings. There can be no "user's guide" or standard manual for such programs, the cultural sensitivity they require, and their practical ethics. This makes the role of counselors and other professionals involved in such programs ever more complex and difficult.

The Book's Composition

Following the introduction, the first chapter presents the rationale, role and dilemmas of genetic counseling. I discuss the ethical code of the profession of genetic counseling and the dilemmas inherent in its practice. The literature review is spread throughout this chapter, rather than being concentrated in one part of it. This is because each of the chapter's sections has its own characteristic literature. I engage in each of the respective sections with other scholars who have studied the ideology and practice of genetic counseling, its uptake and outcomes, policy-related and bioethical issues, as well as clients' attitudes. I also discuss the concept of genetic counseling in the community by surveying other community-based programs, with an emphasis on the linkage between consanguinity and genetic screening. I then focus on genetic counseling for inherited hearing loss and thalassemia as representing two concepts of "genetic community." The final section, entitled "genetic counseling as an arena for symbolic interaction," focuses on other (perhaps more conventional) ways of understanding genetic counseling, and explains the analytical novelty of this study.

The broader socio-cultural and political characteristics of Bedouin-Israeli relations provide an important context for considering genetic counseling as an arena for symbolic interaction. This context is introduced at the end of chapter one, and continued more specifically in chapter two, entitled "the setting." While the program reflected a biomedical rationale related to preventive medicine, the condition it tested for—hearing impairment—was a relatively mild disease that for many Bedouin (or western people for that matter) would not entail abortion. Chapter two considers the social construction of hearing loss in the Bedouin community. Clan members increasingly perceived hearing impairments as a disadvantage, even if not a stigma. Hearing-impaired people were likely to have difficulties finding and keeping a job and hearing-impaired women were likely to be married within the family as second, rather than first wives. This chapter also contains a methodological section where the combined methodology (qualitative and quantitative) of the study is explained. In a section entitled "ethnographic reflection" I reflect on the dialectics of researching and intervening as manifested in this study.

The third chapter focuses on the genetic counselors' espoused ideology and practice, and the ethical dilemmas raised by the program. Three major ethical dilemmas are defined and discussed. First, carrier matching raises ethical questions regarding the seeming violation of the patient's lawful right to obtain information about him- or herself. Second, nondirectiveness and patient's autonomy are seemingly compromised by a scheme in which two carriers can be termed "genetically incompatible." Third, the program is ethically questioned by the fact that hearing loss is not a severe disease. These dilemmas do not have clear-cut solutions but rather represent a gray area in which ethical principles acquire new, situated meanings.

The analysis is based on in-depth interviews conducted with counselors and other staff members. A special section is dedicated to the views of Bedouin health professionals, some of whom trained to work as community-outreach assistants in the genetics program.

Chapter four provides baseline information regarding the population in terms of socio-economic status, education, religion, and susceptibility. It then focuses on instruction and counseling sessions as well as interviews with community members. The final section focuses on attitudes of Bedouin women, especially in regard to etiology and heredity, carrier matching, and the issue of abortion.

Counseling does not constitute the only criterion of success since the program aims for a long-term change of attitudes, particularly in regard to the younger generation. The means of re-socialization include school curricula (on human genetics) and a special Arabic-speaking documentary drama, called "Āysha," that was produced especially for the program and has been shown to Bedouin pupils. The former is discussed in chapter five and the latter in chapter six. Chapter five draws on a questionnaire presented to Bedouin teachers and pupils in order to analyze their knowledge of genetics and attitudes towards genetic counseling. Chapter six discusses the educational film, 'Āysha', in which professional actors and "authentic" Bedouin play the fictive story of a young Bedouin girl from a family with a genetic disease, who is destined by her father to marry her cousin against her will. Following a genetic test in which she and her cousin are found to be carriers, she breaks the match and finally marries a suitor from a different tribe. This film epitomizes the program's rationale by purporting to translate medical terms and thinking into local cultural terms and speak to local customs such as the Muslim ban on abortion and agnatic consanguinity. I use a textual analysis of the film's changing script versions to demonstrate its inherent dilemmas and how it offered to solve them. In addition, focus groups conducted with Bedouin teachers and pupils are used to assess their interpretation of and attitudes towards the film and its themes. This chapter concludes with questionnaire data on the different interpretations of nondirectiveness in genetic counseling by Bedouin and Jewish students.

* * *

The experimental program for carrier-matching studied here presents a complex interface between public and private, professional and lay, modern and traditional dimensions of life. As can be expected in a cross-cultural intervention program, this interface was not without breaches and mismatches. These, however, also serve to highlight the negotiated aspects of the medicalization process. "Medicalization" is usually used in a critical manner that assumes a dominant and homogenous biomedical narrative enforced by paternalistic professionals on passive patients. The findings presented here challenge this premise.

The relationship between the new genetics and medicalization has been studied mainly in terms of the medicalization of deviance (e.g., homosexuality, aggression, and mental illness) and the potential impact of behavioral genetics on the medicalization process. In focusing on genetic counseling, this study extends the scope of the discussion to include the medicalization of normal life processes such as match-making and family-planning. Following the sequencing of the mutation and the launching of the program for carrier matching, a re-definition of social reality was gradually taking place in the targeted Bedouin populations.

While the program was well intended, its design and implementation raised quite a few ethical dilemmas, which had no clear-cut answers. As the program was put in motion, the dilemmas—in a manner typical of organizational dynamics—were gradually submerged by the argument of cultural adaptation. In this manner, the directive use of "genetic compatibility" for carrier matching was justified as an adaptation to the constraints presented by local religion (the ban on abortion) and local norms (preferred patrilateral parallel cousin marriage). In effect, however, a kind of reverse "cultural adaptation" also occurred in which some of the Bedouin who used the program adapted its counseling to suit their own interests (which were quite different from the program's goals).

By bringing in the agendas of community members, this study also shows that the "patients" are not necessarily passive. Furthermore, medicalization is not a dichotomous process that engenders either compliance or resistance. Rather, the process of medicalization can entail a multiplicity of non-compliant utilization strategies. Such individual agendas were not disclosed in counseling and could be uncovered only through personal interviews with counselees. The public format of the counseling session leaves little elbowroom for outspoken negotiation. The result was a separation between the public discourse of counseling and the private realms of attitudes and decision-making. Yet like any medical encounter, counseling does not occur in a vacuum. When used, it always becomes entangled in people's life, and their interests and constraints shape its outcomes. This assertion should serve as a point of departure for the ensuing study.

The Gene and the Genie

Chapter 1

The Rationale, Role and Dilemmas of Genetic Counseling

Genetic counseling was created in order to provide individuals with understandable medical information concerning genetic diseases, for example whether a fetus is affected or whether a person is a carrier. It is defined as "an educational process that seeks to assist affected and/or at-risk individuals to understand the nature of the genetic disorder, its transmission, and the options open to them in management and family planning" (Kelly, 1986: 343). There are already quite a few types of counseling. I use the term genetic *counseling* as an umbrella concept encompassing all types of genetic screening and testing. Genetic *screening* refers to genetic tests carried out on a population as a whole and where, originally, there is no previous suspicion of a genetic condition. Genetic *testing* is used to diagnose a genetic condition in an individual or several members of a family, when there is usually a suspicion of a genetic condition. Genetic screening, in contrast to testing, is usually not initiated by the individual who is its subject but by the provider of the screening service.

One of the most common types of genetic counseling is the prenatal testing of fetuses. There are currently two established forms of prenatal tests—amniocentesis and chorionic villus DNA sampling (CVS, for short). Genetic testing is also commonly conducted in the context of newborn (or neonatal) screening. Neonatal screening is of particular value for diseases in which early prophylaxis or treatment is of value, sickle cell anemia and phenylketonuria, for example.

Another common type of testing is individual carrier testing. Carrier testing is done for recessive disorders like thalassemia and Tay-Sachs disease. The most common form is individual carrier testing. Some screening programs that are aimed at couples rather than individuals use stepwise testing. In stepwise testing, one of the partners is tested first. If s/he is a carrier, the other partner is also tested, since the couple risks having an affected child only if both parents are carriers. Carrier matching is yet another form of testing that matches the carrier status of two partners. A match is considered "genetically incompatible" only if the two partners are carriers. Another form of testing called predictive counseling tests the individual for late-onset conditions such as Huntington's disease, or for pre-dispositional conditions like familial breast cancer.

Screening for genetic variants that predispose individuals or their offspring to disease may be performed at the general population level or may instead be targeted at the relatives of previously identified carriers. The latter strategy, most intensively assessed for cystic fibrosis, has come to be known as "cascade genetic screening" (Krawczak et al., 2001). Finally, as more experience is gained of preimplantation diagnosis, that is DNA-based analysis of a few cells of fertilized ova obtained by in vitro fertilization, this is likely to become the method of choice for many couples at risk for having a child with a serious genetic disease. Preimplantation counseling has the particular advantage of removing the need for termination of pregnancy.

Social dilemmas are found in nearly all aspects of genetic counseling, such as deciding when and where to administer genetic screening, how to assure participation, compliance and quality control, and how to use, disclose, store and control genetic information (Holtzman and Shapiro, 1998; Wertz and Fletcher, 1989). Having an interest in minimizing the burden illness imposes on those who pay taxes, the state may take a far more involved stance toward influencing reproductive decisions through mandating specific genetic tests. Research that associates race or ethnicity with a genetic disposition to disease (e.g., sickle-cell anemia and African-Americans, or Tay-Sachs and Ashkenazi Jews) presents risks of group discrimination and stigmatization (King, 1992). Some have proposed that communities should have the authority to approve or veto genetic research involving their members (Sharp and Foster, 2000). Indeed, many communities have traditional norms and values that are incongruent with the "standard view" of genetic counseling (Christakis, 1992; Foster et al., 1998; Chadwick et al., 1999).

Perspectives on Nondirectiveness versus Eugenics

Institutional pressures to lower health-care costs remain a stimulus to the eugenic approach inherent in genetic counseling. At the same time, genetic counseling must remain nondirective for the sake of individual autonomy. The latter ideology has led, in the West, to the development of universal and standard criteria such as informed consent, nondirectiveness, and autonomy.[2] In the US, a President's Commission (1983: 13) described the counseling process as "attempting to achieve non-directiveness and avoiding all value preference." The National Society of Genetic Counselors (1997) in the US similarly described counseling as based on offering support and respect for the counselee's decisions. The Society's brochure also contains the following claim:

> MYTH: Genetic counselors tell people what decisions to make.
> FACT: Genetic counselors encourage people to make decisions that reflect their own personal and cultural beliefs, values and goals. Genetic counselors support the decisions made by couples and individuals.

Originating from the writings of Carl Rogers on client-centered therapy, nondirectiveness is widely understood to mean that counseling should be client-led (Pilnick, 2002). The ethos of genetic counseling is hence for the client to set the agenda; the first element of genetic counseling should be listening (Clark et al., 1996). In practice, however, genetic counselors continue to play the role of both information-providers and advisers. The norm of nondirectiveness may have been introduced to correct the historical misuse of eugenics, but in effect genetic counseling is inherently prescriptive (Chadwick, 1998; Resta, 1997; Wertz and Fletcher, 1989). The agendas of counselors and counselees are frequently discordant (Kessler, 1992). Many times, counselees simply lack the knowledge or assertiveness to make their agenda heard.

The basic dilemma of genetic counseling, then, can be described in the following manner. On the one hand, the goal of reducing the prevalence of genetic diseases has been supported through a functionalist approach stressing utilitarian ethics (e.g., the moral obligation to reach the greatest happiness of the greatest number of people). On the other hand, the "standard view" (at least in the West) of genetic counseling is based on liberal ethics that give precedence to individual variation and autonomy.

The prominent Western stance views eugenics as a morally negative, coercive social program enforced by the state (Kevles, 1985). A question posed by many geneticists is whether we should denounce each and every form of eugenic thought and practice because of its horrendous misuses by the state in the past (Caplan, McGee & Magnus, 1999). A complementary question is whether avoiding eugenics in genetic counseling is actually tenable. In a

2. See, e.g., the general guidelines for genetic testing that have been issued by the NIH (1997); or the NAS (1975) early report, where ethical aspects are presented from the view of a "perfect" screener. However, many leaders of American genetics also made contradictory eugenic statements (Resta, 1997).

recent worldwide survey of genetics professionals, the word "eugenics" was avoided but questions were asked about the perceived goals of genetics (Wertz, 1998). The majority of geneticists in 12 out of the 36 nations surveyed (but not in the US) agreed with the statement: "An important goal of genetic counseling is to reduce the number of deleterious genes in the population."[3] Wertz (1998) also found that most genetic counseling around the world is directive, and that the "nondirective counseling" found in English-speaking countries is actually an aberration from the general practice of giving advice.

Farrel et al. (2001) who studied the differences between newborn screening programs in the US, report that when professionals were asked about directive and nondirective counseling techniques, responses were mixed. Some respondents said that they often use directive counseling to advise against subsequent pregnancies, while others were more nondirective and avoided definite recommendations about the next pregnancy. Furthermore, the authors were struck by the large number of respondents agreeing with the statement about the "suitability for reproduction" of the patient. During development of their survey, the authors included this wording with the expectation that most respondents would disagree with the phrasing as it was reminiscent of eugenics.

In sum, the intention of genetic counseling, on both the community and the individual level, is eugenicist by implication.[4] Governmental pressures to lower health-care costs remain a stimulus to eugenic approaches. Critics of geneticization have argued that eugenics is built into genetic counseling because of the normativity of medicine. Ten Have (2000) argued that the norm of nondirectiveness in human genetics may have been introduced against the historical misuse of eugenics, but in effect genetic counseling is inherently prescriptive. Indeed, analysis of actual genetic counseling sessions indicates that nondirectiveness, in the sense that the counselor withholds advice or judgment, is seldom accomplished (Michie et al., 1997), and that the mechanism of informed consent does not work in reality (Dunne & Warren, 1998). These studies were conducted in the US, and not in developing countries. Directiveness also creeps in when providers are *mandated* to offer prenatal screening, as is the case in California for screening for neural tube

3. Note that when a slightly different phrasing was used, i.e., "prevention of diseases is a highly important goal of genetic counseling," 52 per cent of the surveyed North-American genetic counselors also agreed (Wertz & Fletcher, 1989).

4. Holtzman (1998) argues that prenatal diagnosis followed by selective abortion has replaced sterilization as "the major eugenic technique."

defects and Down syndrome (Press and Browner, 1993). Importantly, counselees are considerably critical of nondirectiveness as an ideal, and often perceive nondirectiveness as an attempt to "hide something" (Shiloh, 1996).

Genetic Counseling and Medicalization

The hegemony of biomedical culture has generated a process sociologists termed as medicalization, meaning that more and more of human behavior is being defined as a medical problem, hence mandating or licensing the medical profession to provide some type of treatment for it (Zola, 1972; Conrad, 1975, 1992; Illich, 1976). Medicalization has occurred in broad areas of human life such as deviance (alcoholism, mental disorders, eating disorders, learning disabilities etc.), as well as in common life processes including childbirth, aging, menstruation, menopause, infertility, anxiety, and death. The advent of genetic research, testing and counseling can be seen as furthering the medicalization of human life. Generally speaking, genetics has become an explanatory frame for a wide range of human problems, positing that genes are a key component in producing particular diseases or behaviors (Conrad, 1997, 1999). To this trend belong popular discussions of "the gene for schizophrenia," "the gene for alcoholism" or "the gene for homosexuality."

Members of disability rights movements have raised another form of criticism against genetic screening programs, which is connected to the general argument regarding medicalization as well as to the eugenic aspects of genetic counseling discussed in the previous section (Parens and Asch, 2000). Some disability rights scholars argue that prenatal genetic testing does not share the traditional medical goal of preventing or treating disease in individuals, but instead seeks to prevent the existence of people with disabilities. Genetic screening is typically done with the goal of identifying potential parents at risk of genetically passing on serious disease, or identifying an affected fetus so that the pregnancy can be terminated. This is criticized as eugenic. As Tom Shakespeare, a disability rights activist and sociologist, has written:

> The Human Genome Project has been hailed as the Holy Grail of future health. I would argue that it does not mark a radical departure from traditional approaches to the 'disability problem'. While historical genetics operates at the level of populations, contemporary eugenics operates at the level of individuals and families. While the rhetoric speaks of improving health, the current reality is that detection and termination are the only option in most cases (Shakespeare, 1995: 8).

The traditional argument against this criticism claims that the desirability of preventing serious genetically transmitted disabilities has no implications for how people with those disabilities can or should be treated, and, in particular, does not justify their mistreatment in any way (WHO, 2002). While the validity of this argument should be empirically tested, it also has theoretical problems. For example, who can or should define which diseases are severe enough to justify screening? Severity is a subjective term, influenced by expectations and norms. Only a very few genetic disorders, such as Lesch-Nyhan or Tay-Sachs disease, are so severe as to make the lives of people who have them perhaps not worth living. The vast majority of conditions for which genetic testing is now and will, in the future, be possible are not so severe; they leave an affected individual with a life that from the individual's perspective is clearly worth living.

My use of the term "medicalization" implies a system of control and surveillance. The relationship between the new genetics and medicalization, which has been studied mainly in the context of deviance, is still an open issue. Here I focus on genetic counseling and the medicalization of normal life processes such as match-making and family-planning. The genetics program offered to the Bedouin was also a context for the social construction of a new reality, where medical concepts of genetic risk were blended with local norms and beliefs. Traditional patterns of behavior such as match-making were put under medical surveillance. Congenital hearing loss, a common condition in the community that was largely a part of its normative social reality, increasingly became a source of potential stigma and labeling. By focusing on a relatively non-severe condition such as congenital hearing loss, the case for medicalization can be more clearly made.

Medicalization is usually used in a critical manner (i.e., "overmedicalization") that assumes a dominant and homogenous biomedical narrative enforced on passive patients. This study provides a context for challenging this conception. I am interested in asking whether medicalization implies complete compliance on the part of both patients and professionals, and what hybrid strategies can be found when we move beyond the dichotomy of compliance versus resistance. For this purpose I focus on the genetics program as a locus of negotiation where multiple 'definitions of the situation' are constructed, exchanged, and challenged.

Geneticization and Public Policy

I use the term "geneticization"—originally coined by Lippman (1992)—as an umbrella concept for the various implications and practices of human genetics, such as education, public imagery, screening, testing, and counseling. Ideologies of geneticization, as we saw, are split between neutrality, nondirectiveness, and patient's autonomy—and, on the opposite side, eugenics and paternalism. Recent advances in genetics and especially the completion of the Human Genome Project will continue to increase the practice of genetic testing and counseling in areas such as late-onset and multifactorial disorders, susceptibility conditions, and single nucleotide polymorphism (Mahowald et al., 1998).

Social and ethical dilemmas are combined with public policy issues in nearly all stages of the genetic counseling procedure, such as deciding when and where to administer genetic screening, how to assure participation, compliance and quality control, and how to use, disclose, store and control genetic information (Holtzman and Shapiro, 1998; Khoury et al., 2000). In the US, genetic discrimination by federal employers was outlawed under the Clinton administration and the Genetic Nondiscrimination in Health Insurance and Employment Act of 1999 would extend this protection to the private sector. Another issue is public participation in policy making: despite their public relevance, key federal advisory committees making policy recommendations regarding human genetics are staffed mainly by representatives of academia and industry (Ard and Natowicz, 2001).

Specific public policy issues in genetic counseling and testing, that also carry social and ethical dilemmas, include the following (see also Wertz and Fletcher, 1989):

1. Whether and how to provide fairer access to existing genetic services;
2. Whether to test children under 18 with the informed consent of their parents, and whether to disclose the child's carrier status to his parents;
3. Whether to protect the choice of abortion for genetic reasons or the choice not to abort, where either of these choices is under attack, and whether to establish a choice to abort for genetic reasons where such a choice does not yet exist;
4. Whether to screen targeted populations, thus potentially generating (or increasing) ethnic and social stigmatization;
5. Whether access to personal genetic information should be kept from employers or insurers, to prevent genetic discrimination.
6. Whether full disclosure is necessary because of the patient's "right to know", or should it be left to professional judgement;
7. Whether the use of prenatal diagnosis for sex selection should be ruled out;
8. Whether directive genetic counseling should be part of public policy in cases of high genetic risk and parental incapacity.

While genetic counseling has been created for individual purposes, in reality it also involves the spouse, the family, and the community. To date, policy frameworks for genetic research have focused on perceived benefits and risks of the individual. Little mention was made of possible group benefits or risks. The individual level, which concerns the patient-counselor interaction, often depends on community-level norms such as consanguinity or banning of selective abortion. In trying to find a point of convergence for this broad list of dilemmas, my focus will be on studying the expressions of these dilemmas within community-based genetic counseling. My intention is to start with the broad framework of the community and then focus on its interplay with (individual) concepts such as patient's autonomy and informed consent.

Genetic Counseling in the Community

We need to embed analyses of genetic counseling within local communities rather than concentrating on two-person interaction. The individual level, which concerns the patient-counselor interaction, often depends on community-level norms such as patriarchy, consanguinity, or religious banning of abortion. The need for such "community genetics" was raised about 15 years ago, as with the World Health Organization (WHO, 1985) program on thalassemia. However, for many people and organizations the linkage between genetics and community is still a new concept, yet to be defined (Brisson, 2000).

Some have proposed supplemental community-based reviews of research on genetic differences between populations (Sharp and Foster, 2000). In contrast to this position, critics have focused almost entirely on group consent—the idea that communities should have the authority to approve or veto research involving their members. We need to be able to move beyond this debate by exploring the process of genetic counseling in the community as an arena for negotiation. Such a focus, as I will later show, can go beyond dichotomies of "group consent/veto" and explore the diverse strategies employed by community members and professionals.

Models of Community-Based Programs for Genetic Counseling

Cross-cultural genetics programs implemented in immigrant communities have usually succeeded in increasing the uptake of genetic services while at the same time increasing the awareness of cultural, social and economic differences (Weil, 2001; Mittman et al., 1998). These genetics programs also highlight the risk of coercion. Experience in a number of countries has already demonstrated the potential for coercive pressures from government and society in top-down genetic screening and testing programs. For example, in some countries it is now mandatory to have a test for thalassemia before getting married (WHO, 1997). These cases highlight the need to carefully design such interventions. In addition to a strong emphasis on education and engagement, community-based genetic services should offer several options for premarital as well as prenatal testing.

Carrier testing or screening of individual or married couples, rather than premarital "carrier matching," is the more common counseling style in the West. Most of the data on motives for participation have been obtained from programs offering carrier screening during pregnancy (Kaback et al., 1974; Mennie et al., 1993; Miadzybrodzka et al., 1995; Grody et al., 1997; Model et al., 2000). It was found that the decision to participate was mostly made by women, who were often initially tested without discussing it with their partner. Anxiety has been reported among those who are tested positive, while waiting for their partner's results. Offering carrier screening outside pregnancy shows low participation rates when no pregnancy is planned, but interest is higher when there are plans for having children (on preconceptional counseling see Honnor et al., 2000; Henneman et al., 2001). Genetic screening programs that take advantage of community engagement have been successful in reducing the prevalence of birth defects and genetic diseases, for example in Sardinia and Cyprus (Cao et al., 1989; Angastiniotis and Hadjiminas, 1981) and among orthodox Ashkenazi Jews (Mertz, 1987; Abeliovich et al., 1996; Broide et al., 1993). Relatively high levels of consanguinity characterize these populations.

The Bedouin populations studied here were at risk for thalassemia and congenital hearing loss (or NSRD, Non-Syndromic Recessive Deafness, in the professional jargon).[5] The two conditions—NSRD and thalassemia—represent different paradigms in terms of the disease, its severity and social construction, and the cultural aspects of the at-risk community where the disease is prevalent.

---

5. I am aware that many hearing-impaired people would take issue with the use of words like "deaf" and "deafness." Where the text is mine, I have used "hearing impairment" instead of "deafness" to denote hearing loss which may range from mild to profound and may be sensorineural, conductive, or mixed. However, the term "Deaf" is used to denote cultural deafness. Where I am using accepted medical acronyms (e.g. NSRD) or quoting, I have remained loyal to the original use of words.

Genetic Counseling for Inherited Hearing Loss and Thalassemia: Two Concepts of "Genetic Community"

The ensuing comparison focuses on the cultural aspects of inherited hearing loss and thalassemia rather than on their (evidently different) clinical symptoms, etiology and treatment. Thalassemia and inherited hearing loss present two different kinds of "genetic communities." This difference is based on variations in the concept of culture. "Culture" can be described as *geographical* (e.g., European culture), *ethnic* (e.g., Latino, African American), *ability-related* (e.g., Deaf Culture) and *traditional* (e.g., Chinese culture of Asian immigrants in the US). Each of these categories, although they can be inter-connected, has its own unique issues and dynamics (Johnson, 1990). In our case, "genetic communities" that are at-risk for thalassemia, belong primarily to the *ethnic* and *geographical* cultural categories, while inherited hearing loss is a clear example of the *ability* category.

The hemoglobinopathies (thalassemias, sickle cell disease and variants) have a particularly high frequency in sub-Saharan Africa, the Mediterranean region, the Middle East, the Indian subcontinent and throughout southeast Asia (Cao et al., 1997; WHO, 2002: 44). The control and management of these disorders is now well-established in some developed countries but thousands of children are dying from these conditions in poorer parts of the world. Furthermore, because these are genetic disorders and there is no definitive cure for any of them, and this is likely to be the case for the foreseeable future, they require a lifetime of medical treatment. The severe forms of disease require lifelong transfusion and expensive drugs for removing iron that accumulates in multi-transfused children. Life expectancy with such management extends into the third decade (Cao et al., 1997). Many countries have thus opted for prenatal screening and, if parents find it acceptable, prenatal diagnosis and termination of pregnancy if the fetus is affected (WHO, 2002). An emerging alternative to this traditional management is bone marrow transplantation from siblings. With this procedure the estimates for disease-free survival are 90% to 95% among patients at low risk (Cao et al., 1997). However, this procedure is very expensive, about 50,000 USD, and requires special medical expertise and technology.

Genetic counseling for thalassemia belongs to a category where the genetic community is formed around kinship (consanguinity is usually prevalent) and distinct ethnic characteristics. The characteristics of kinship, consanguinity, and ethnicity are often highlighted by the counseling programs targeting specific at-risk populations. For example, the "Cyprus screening program," with its Church-mandated marriage certificate, has become a context for genetic services provided for the Greek-Orthodox population in Cyprus. Another community-based counseling program is similarly connected with the British Pakistani community (Darr, 1996). These populations, with their distinct ethnic and cultural characteristics, obviously exist independently of the disease. The counseling programs developed by and for these populations therefore highlight characteristics of an existing sociocultural reality.

In contrast, the cultural aspects surrounding inherited hearing loss belong to the category of *ability*. It has been estimated that about 1 in 1,000 births is affected by hearing loss, with roughly half due to genetic etiology (McKusick, 1990). Although genetic counseling for hearing-impaired individuals and their families has been available for a long time (Nance, 1971,1977), many hearing-impaired adults do not seek genetic services due in part to the communicational and cultural differences of this group (Israel et al., 1992). Indeed, within Deaf culture (spelled with an uppercase 'D'), deafness may not be regarded as a 'disability' but a cultural difference that does not require genetic screening (Padden and Humphries, 1988). Many Deaf people marry another deaf person and many feel that it would be more desirable to have deaf children (Bienvenu and Colonomus, 1985). In contrast, there may be ethno-cultural communities where congenital hearing loss is considered a burden, a handicap and a stigma. In other words, there can be various combinations within the cultural matrix of geography, ethnicity, tradition, and ability.

Many genetic centers around the world now offer genetic testing for mutations in the gene coding for the protein Connexin 26, thought to be the most common cause of congenital hearing loss (Cohn and Kelly, 1999). Unlike thalassemia, congenital hearing loss can be perceived in different ways. The "medical model" views it as a pathology to be treated or cured, whereas the "cultural model" (developed in the US) sees it as a condition to be understood and preserved (Arnos et al., 1991). In a UK survey conducted by Middleton et al. (2001), it was found that hearing individuals with a family history of congenital hearing loss were more likely to be interested in using prenatal testing for this condition. Culturally Deaf individuals were the least likely to be interested in prenatal testing. Most participants from all groups said they would not act on the results of a prenatal genetic test. The majority said they would only have prenatal diagnosis in order to prepare for the language needs of the child. The possibility of terminating the pregnancy of a hearing-impaired fetus raises the ethical question of when an abortion is ethically justified, something which has been largely put aside in discussing the termination of pregnancy due to thalassemia. The decision to perform prenatal testing for non-severe genetic conditions such as congenital hearing loss relies on the discretion of the individual clinician. Middleton et al. (2001) report that 9% of British and 35% of American genetics professionals would perform prenatal diagnosis for a hearing-impaired couple wanting to have hearing-impaired children. Obviously, there is no consensus on the subject.

Consanguinity and Genetic Counseling

The term 'consanguineous' literally means related by blood, so consanguineous marriages are defined as marriages between blood relatives. For practical purposes, geneticists usually classify unions between second cousins or closer as consanguineous, because the genetic risk for less closely related couples differs only marginally from that in non-consanguineous unions. In the countries of the Eastern Mediterranean Region, consanguineous marriage is common in Muslim as well as some Christian and Jewish communities. While in general use 'consanguinity' simply means some degree of recognized relatedness by 'blood,' I use the term more specifically to refer to rates of shared consanguinity resulting from parallel cousin marriage and, in general, group endogamy.

In the mainly Muslim countries of the Eastern Mediterranean region, and in most parts of south Asia, consanguineous marriage accounts for from 20% to over 50% of the total in the present generation (WHO, 1997). On average, first cousins inherit one quarter of their genes from each of their common grandparents, and one eighth of their genes are identical by inheritance. The children of first cousin parents inherit identical gene copies from each parent at one sixteenth (6.25%) of all gene loci, over and above the baseline level of homozygosity in the general population. Double first cousin marriages, where the spouses have both sets of grandparents in common, also occur. Here 12.5% of the children's gene pairs are likely to be identical by descent. Consanguineous marriage does not significantly affect the frequency of characteristics that derive from dominant alleles, since these are expressed independently of the genetic make-up of the partner. It is generally considered to play a minor role in multifactorial inheritance, although the extent of any effect remains to be clarified. It definitely increases the likelihood that characteristics that derive from recessive alleles will be expressed in the offspring because related partners inherit a significant number of identical genes from their common ancestor(s), which may then be passed on to their children in the homozygous state. Examples of congenital disorders that are more common when the parents are related include forms of mental retardation, blindness and deafness, and common disorders like beta-thalassemia in Cyprus or sickle cell trait in eastern Saudi Arabia. Therefore, where consanguineous marriage is customary, an increased birth prevalence of some types of congenital malformation, deafness and mental handicap is to be anticipated.

Some three decades ago it was predicted that with industrialization, greater population mobility, a decline in family size, and higher literacy rates, there would be a rapid reduction in the prevalence of consanguineous marriage (Haldane, 1963). Haldane's prediction has largely come to pass, especially in industrialized and rapidly urbanizing societies. In some areas, this prediction failed owing to the cultural significance of consanguinity and the persistence of tradition. Among communities in the Eastern Mediterranean Region in which cousin marriage is preferred, the highest rates are consistently reported in the more traditional rural areas (Bittles, 1992). Cousin marriage is also most prevalent among the poorer and less educated sections of Muslim society and among couples marrying for the first time (WHO, 1997). The change predicted by Haldane and other propagators of modernization should therefore take place in its own time and any effort to hasten it for genetic reasons may be harmful, especially for the less advantaged members of society. Indeed, the loosening of family ties is one of the major social problems of more developed societies.

Despite being often cited as a religious norm, cousin marriage has no Muslim basis. Although Islam neither forbids nor prescribes this particular type of marriage (Abd Al-Ati, 1995:136), the *Quran* cites the prophet as commanding people to "marry those who are distant." The strengthening of family ties and the maintenance of family property are usually major considerations in choosing a cousin marriage (Bittles et al., 1991; Khlat, 1988). Marriage with a relative is also preferred because of the comparative ease with which premarital negotiations can be conducted, and because it is considered to be favorable for the woman's status. In many communities where cousin marriage is common, the family name and property are inherited through the male line (descent is patrilineal), the men and their descendants tending to stay together, especially when the family owns land. At marriage, a woman leaves her own family to enter her husband's family. Cousin marriage often softens the implications of this transition.

On first considering the facts, it often seems that affected births can be prevented if couples at risk are identified prior to marriage, on the assumption that they will then decide to separate and each find another, non-carrier partner. This argument brings together the issues of consanguinity and community-based genetic counseling, and has been quite pertinent in the context of thalassemia. However, we understand too little of how most marriages come about to make any valid assumptions about the effect of genetic information on choice of partner. In all societies, marriage is a complex social phenomenon that involves many family members besides the prospective couple, and partners are usually selected because of a strong personal preference, for valid family reasons or for traditional reasons, or a combination of all three.

Before prenatal diagnosis was feasible, a research study of the effect on choice of marriage partner of informing young people and their families of their carrier status was carried out in the Arta area of Greece, where 20% of the population carry either thalassemia or sickle cell allele. All young people of marriageable age were screened and counseled, and counseling contact was maintained for a two-year period. When the pattern of marriages was assessed at the end of this period, screening had had no measurable effect on choice of partner (Stamatoyannopoulos, 1974).

The evolution of thalassemia screening in Cyprus is perhaps the most well-documented example of its kind. This condition was not identified in the island until 1944, when, after a major malaria eradication program and accompanying improvements in public health, it became clear that among the children there was a common form of anemia, which was later identified as thalassemia. By the early 1970's it was estimated that, if no steps were taken to control the disease, in about 40 years time the blood required to treat all the severely affected children would amount to 78,000 units per annum, 40% of the population would have to be blood donors, and the total cost of managing the disease would equal or exceed the Island's health budget.

In the 70s carrier matching began in Cyprus, with the emphasis that marriages between carriers were actively discouraged. This proved unacceptable to the population and was soon abandoned "because of evasions" (Angastiniotis and Hadjiminas, 1981). Once prenatal diagnosis became possible for thalassemia it was made available within the Cypriot health service and confidential premarital screening was mandated. It was then found that 98% of couples at risk detected prior to marriage proceeded to marry, even though Cypriot parents often have considerable influence on choice of partner. Nevertheless, couples used the information on genetic risk in a variety of ways to obtain a healthy family and the annual number of new births of thalassemic children has fallen almost to zero in Cyprus. Less than 5% of this fall is due to separation of engaged couples, about 80% is due to prenatal diagnosis and selective abortion, and around 20% is because couples at risk have rather fewer children than couples not at risk (Angastiniotis et al., 1986).

Other reports of the Cyprus case, however, present a more complex picture. The introduction of fetal diagnosis in 1981, and of first-trimester diagnosis (i.e., CVS) since 1986, no doubt had a crucial role in reducing the prevalence of thalassemia. However, it should be noted that premarital screening that began as early as 1972 preceded fetal diagnosis and perhaps paved the way for it. Minas Hadjiminas (1994: 36), a Cypriot doctor and head of the thallasemia Center, who described the program to the Council of Europe on Bioethics, wrote in his report: "I have seen couples coming together to the genetic counseling center with an understanding not to marry if both were carriers. I have seen young ladies who were carriers coming with the would-be husband to be tested with the understanding that they would not marry if he was a carrier." This quote is exceptionally directive and, given the severe price of marriage cancellation, stands in complete opposition to Hadjiminas's observation that "the youngsters come forward with pleasure to have the test and subsequently without any pressure from any quarters make their decision in an atmosphere of friendliness and peace" (1994: 36). Note also that in 1983 (two years after the introduction of prenatal testing), the Cyprus Church (which objects to abortions) introduced a "premarital certificate" mandating that partners are tested before marriage. Lab results were kept confidential as the certificate only stated that the bearer was examined and advised for thalassemia (Ioannou, 1999: 61). This "unusual compliance mechanism" is also obviously directive. All these factors highlight the ethical problem of free choice in a directive environment and of claiming that individuals are "autonomous" whereas the framework for decision-making has already been constructed by health professionals (Hoedemaekers and ten Have, 1998). While illustrating the ethical problems involved in such programs, these factors also indicate the role of premarital screening in the success of the program.

Perhaps the best example of successful community-based premarital carrier screening and matching is *Dor Yeshorim*, the program developed by the orthodox Ashkenazi Jewish community and currently implemented in Israel, the UK, and the US. Established in 1983 in New York by a Rabbi, the program started with Tay-Sachs screening and later added screening for cystic fibrosis and Canavan disease (Mertz, 1987; Abeliovich et al., 1996; Broide et al., 1993). In the orthodox Ashkenazi Jewish community, birth control and abortion are forbidden (unless the woman's life is endangered by her pregnancy); and marriages are pre-arranged through match-making. The program includes premarital carrier testing and confidential storage of the results in a computerized system, which enables future matching of the carrier status of potential mates. Individuals who are carriers but are going to marry a non-carrier never learn their genetic status. In the few cases of "genetic incompatibility" (carrier-by-carrier match) no one besides the close family has to know about it. Using the match-making procedure, the engagement is cancelled at the earliest possible stage. The success of *Dor Yeshorim* results from the relatively large number of severe diseases being tested, the strong support of the religious leaders of the Jewish community, and the familiarity of community members with biomedical technology. The compliance rate with *Dor Yeshorim* is over 90% and in recent years hardly any children affected with Tay-Sachs or cystic fibrosis have been born in this community to couples who married during the last decade (Sagi, 1998: 427). Indeed, Israeli genetic counselor Michal Sagi (1998: 427) concludes her discussion of *Dor Yeshorim* by suggesting that "similar programs should be offered in other communities in which marriages are prearranged and termination of pregnancy is not accepted." An example would be the Bedouin community.

Genetic Counseling as an Arena for Symbolic Interaction

Despite the recognition of genetic counseling as a *process of communication*, centered on the clients and their needs, it has rarely been studied as such. As most studies are centered on outcomes, decision-making and attitudes, what happens within actual counseling sessions largely remains 'a mysterious black box' (Kessler, 1992: 6). Studies of genetic counseling have centered on such issues as outcome and uptake measures (e.g., Watson et al., 1995, 1996; Michie et al., 1997b; Sorenson et al., 1981), impact on reproductive decision making (e.g., Hildes et al., 1993) and client satisfaction (e.g., Bleiker et al., 1997). The theorizing and measurement of research questions have been largely framed within a positivistic paradigm that entails the use of quantitative methods (Pilnick and Dingwall, 2001). Established psychological scales and questionnaires were used to address specific aspects of counseling such as verbal behavior (Mendez and Shymansky, 1984) and patients' reactions, while borrowing existing social psychology concepts such as family systems (Eunpu, 1997; Kessler and Bloch, 1998), depression (McConkie-Russel and Sullivan, 1999; Lerman et al., 1997, 1998), and perceived personal control (Berkenstadt et al., 1999). Some researchers of genetic counseling have recently stressed the benefit of adding qualitative methods to the dominant framework of quantitative studies (e.g., conversation analysis in Pilnick, 2002; grounded theory in McAllister, 2001, 1999 and Michie et al., 1996; ethnographic analysis in Chapple and May, 1996; Chapple et al., 1997). This growing corpus of research represents the need to develop evidence-based, grounded theories about the processes going in and around genetic counseling. McAllister (2001: 235), for example, advocates the qualitative-interpretive approach as a way to avoid relying on "*a-priori* theorizing that runs the risk of introducing substantial subjective bias."

I employ in this study a symbolic interactionist perspective that provides a middle way between the ideology and practice of genetic counseling. Symbolic interactionism can show us how to go beyond theoretical oppositions that consider ideology and practice as different facets of a pre-conceived, objective social order (see also Wiener, 2000; Gerhardt, 2000; Strauss, 1978, 1993, 1997; Strauss et al., 1997). In my view, a symbolic interactionist point of departure for the study of genetic counseling consists of two premises regarding negotiation. First, it involves focusing on the ways in which ethical considerations involved in genetic counseling acquire situated meanings within institutional and political contexts. Second, it entails realizing the different meanings of genetic counseling for the participants, and the different arenas (public and private) in which these meanings are negotiated.

Studies of genetic counseling, even when focused on biased communication between counselor and counselee, have often ignored the negotiation process. Researching the consultation in isolation tends to neglect those aspects of communication that remain unspoken. Studies have either failed to see how social worlds, which they analyzed, depended on continuous flow of (often tacit) negotiations, or else have disregarded the extent to which social change occurs incessantly in the wake of unrelenting negotiative re-arrangements between actors. Symbolic interactionism can tell us more about genetic counseling by applying the "negotiation paradigm." As Strauss (1978: 98–99) put it,

> "The key terms of the paradigm and their use in the case analyses are as follows. First, the negotiations themselves will be described [....] Included in the descriptions will be the accompanying interactions, types of actors, their strategies and tactics, some consequences of the negotiations, and embedded negotiation subprocesses of negotiations; for example, making trade-offs, obtaining kickbacks, paying off debts, and negotiating agreements. Second, the structural context is that within which the negotiations take place, in the larger sense. For each case of negotiation, it will be necessary to bring out some of the salient structural properties that bear on the negotiation."

The counseling session should therefore be understood according to the "definitions of the situation" held by the various participants. As Rapp (1999) points out in her anthropological study of amniocentesis, we should be particularly attentive to the ways these genetic testing technologies become signifiers of "scientific literacy" and social status. Through their use of these genetic technologies, women and men are forced, as Rapp argues, "to judge the quality of their own fetuses, making concrete and embodied decisions about the standards for entry into the human community" (1999: 3). While counselees can acquire a commonality of perspective with counselors by learning and developing together the symbols by which aspects of the world are identified, still many would define the situation in quite different terms. The communication of genetic risk, for example, requires that counselors translate statistical and biomedical knowledge into more familiar notions. Rapp notes that although such "translation" existed in the New York hospitals she studied, it also rewarded "middle" strata compliance and reproduced the disadvantaged position of less-educated "nonscience speakers" (1999: 66) by holding them to a level of comprehension that may challenge a truly "informed" decision about amniocentesis. Indeed, establishing a consensus between client and counselor may be impossible given cultural differences in understandings of disability, genetic inheritance, and medical compliance.

In the genetic counseling program studied here, as in many others, a common "lingua franca" or interface culture has developed in the session, since counselors felt that their message was conveyed and counselees could interpret the test results and make use of them. For an outsider, this would gradually assume the appearance of objective reality. In practice, however, participants have different and often conflicting perspectives.

A symbolic interactionist perspective is thus a-priori critical of the management of "nondirectiveness" in any communication process. If a client does not know what will be considered relevant by the counselor, or does not have sufficient background knowledge to formulate appropriate questions, the goal of nondirective (or client-led) counseling becomes interactionally unachievable. In addition, competing perspectives between spouses, parents, or family members are also potentially important. As Pilnick (2002: 85) comments, "if a consultation is to be client-led, the existence of multiple clients raises the question: by which client?" Such considerations underlie the need for more research on the actual process of counseling as symbolic interaction. This includes the individual level (counselor-counselee), the family level, and the communal-social level (Bedouin-Israeli, in our case).

Genetic Counseling in the Socio-Cultural Context of Bedouin-Israeli Relations

Generally speaking, genetic counseling to non-western traditional communities is also a case of "glocalization" (see Raz, 1999)—the interplay between global and local. The "global" is represented by the professional and bioethical mission of genetic counseling, while the "local" consists of the norms and values of the target population. The global-local interplay—a key scenario in contemporary cultural studies (Hannerz, 1992, 1996)—has been traditionally studied either through modernization or world-systems theories. Seen through the mirror of modernization, third-world developing countries (and counselees) are considered to be passively and unreflectively (and often also 'inconsistently') modernized, or acculturated, into Western biomedicine through identical cultural trajectories (Webster, 1984). In this perspective genetic counseling functions as an agent of modernization. On the other hand, genetic counseling could be seen as an agent of eugenics and coerced medicalization. This point of view is usually taken by neo-Marxist analyses such as world-systems theory (Wallerstein, 1974). Concepts such as modernization and world-systems, or acculturation and resistance, are not new in socio-anthropological theory, but their influence is still felt in many contemporary debates. My aim in this study is to take a middle way that can help us move beyond this dichotomy. Despite their theoretical opposition, these perspectives have a common blind spot. They both presume a unilateral structure of Western hegemony whose biomedical culture is imposed on some silent recipient(s). These assumptions about local community passivity have already been refuted by many studies in medical anthropology. Once again, my use of symbolic interactionism in this context is intended to make way for a plurality of 'negotiated meanings' that undermine monolithic narratives of globalization and cultural imperialism. Grounding the practice of genetic counseling within the Bedouin-Israeli context is meant to strengthen the case against community passivity in the face of the medicalization of heredity and reproduction, and to complicate its implications for the analysis of kinship, community, and power relations.

Broader socio-cultural and historical processes of marginalization and state hegemony underpin Bedouin-Jewish relationships in Israel. The Negev Bedouin are a Muslim minority (estimated population around 130,000) residing in the southern part of Israel. In 1998 about 50% of the population lived in seven towns which were planned for them by Israeli governments, while the rest lived in scattered encampments and shantytowns (Annual statistics for 1998). Many Bedouin towns are not self-governed but rather represented by Jewish officials of government Ministries (Dinero, 1998). The formally "unrecognized" villages are denied basic services such as water, electricity, and sewage, and only a few have schools and clinics.

The beginning of this problematic situation can be traced to the 1948 War of Independence, when the Negev area was placed under military administration until 1966. The Bedouin who had remained in the Negev were forcibly moved and confined to a restricted zone in it. The Israeli State expropriated 93% of the Negev area under its Land Acquisition Law, which (following the Ottoman Land Code of 1858) did not recognize Bedouin landholding rights (Jakubovska, 1990; Marks, 1967; Shamir, 1996). The severely diminished area available to the Bedouin marked the end of pastoral nomadism as their primary source of livelihood. Sedenterization of the Bedouin was publicly presented by the Israeli establishment as modernization. Once the military administration was abolished in the Negev, many Bedouin families re-settled the lands they considered theirs by inheritance. These hamlets and encampments were considered illegal by the state. The land dispute has therefore become a perennial source of conflict that underpins Bedouin-Jewish relationships.

While modernization is superficially identified with becoming "more" Israeli, the Bedouin are quite aware of their marginal place in Israeli society. In Bedouin eyes, while the agencies of the Israeli State were concerned with concentrating them in towns, they did little to develop local public services, and less to foster local trade and industry. This led to very high unemployment. According to Marx (2000), the real rate of unemployment among the Bedouin is an estimated 70% (as distinct from the official figure of 25% in Bedouin towns). Conscription to the Israeli military, which is voluntary for the Bedouin and used to be practiced as a means of social mobilization and identification, has dwindled among today's Bedouin youth. On the other hand, the fundamentalist Islamic Movement has become increasingly more popular.

The Bedouin, as Israeli citizens, are entitled for curative health care as promulgated in the National Health Insurance Law of 1995. Genetic counseling services offered to the Bedouin can therefore be seen as a "natural" corollary of the health care they are entitled for. However, this is not so simple. Genetic counseling is also part of the symbolic interactions between Bedouin and Israeli Jews. First of all, community-based genetic counseling such as the one offered to the Bedouin has the potential to stigmatize a population. Such labeling could join, in the case of the Bedouin community, to already existing processes of group position and prejudice. Moreover, issues of family planning and premarital counseling can become very sensitive in the context of national/ethnic conflict. For example, Bedouin individuals could become prejudiced against genetic counseling if they perceive it as an extension of the dominant Israeli establishment and interpret it as an attempt to reduce the birth rate in the Bedouin population.

In the political context of Israeli-Palestinian relations, for example, the notion of "demographic war" looms large. It is a war in which women's bodies are enlisted on both sides in a nationalist struggle to reproduce new citizens. This is evidently a generalization and fieldwork is needed to expose the interplay between nationally-driven pronatalism and individual choices. In a recent anthropological study conducted in an Arab-Israeli village in the Galilee (northern part of Israel), Kanaaneh (2002) argues that among the relatively privileged Palestinians of the Galilee (as opposed to Palestinian populations in the West Bank and Gaza, or to the Bedouin of the Negev), most people are opting for small "high-quality" families, despite their ongoing assertions about the importance of reproducing large "quantities" of Palestinian children, especially sons, who are preferred for the purposes of the national struggle. According to Kanaaneh, this creates tensions of status and identity among Palestinians themselves, as those who use contraception attempt to disassociate themselves from "backward," high-fertility families. It is unclear to what extent the Bedouin identify with the Palestinian uprising (*Intifadah*), and so far there was no Bedouin activity in support of terrorism against Israel. However, the Bedouin are involved in an ethnic conflict with Israel owing to the land problem and a growing social marginalization. After a mass departure to neighboring countries during 1947–1949 (as a result of Israel's War of Independence), the numbers of Negev Bedouin have increased from 12,000 in 1948 to around 130,000 today, forming 24% of the Negev District by the end of 1995 (Borkan et al., 2000). This dramatic natural growth is among the highest in the world. An important factor behind this growth is the Bedouin's high birth rate. In Bedouin society, a large number of children traditionally represented the family's "human resource" and was hence encouraged (a strategy termed "competitive breeding" by Kressel, 1992). Even though shrinking pastoral resources and growing dependency on the Israeli labor market have decreased the material value of children for the nuclear Bedouin family, their socio-political value has been maintained (Meir & Ben-David, 1995). This means that for the Bedouin, too, the politics of reproduction play an important role.

Historically and ideologically, Zionist Israeli society also encouraged pronatalism. This was done as a continuation of the traditional Jewish dictum to "be fruitful and multiply," as well as in the national context of the "demographic threat" posed by the Arabs (Laquer, 1972; Vital, 1975). An average of 4.5 children per family was declared in the 60's as a national priority by Israeli governmental committees established for the encouragement of procreation; pronatalist practices that were implemented for this purpose included state subsidies in areas such as housing mortgage, school tuition, and social security income (Shuval and Anson, 2000: 158-60). Demographic anxiety intensified after the Six Day War of 1967, when Israel conquered a large amount of territory and with it many Palestinians. In parallel to the above-mentioned pronatatlist practices, family planning strategies were downplayed while medical technologies such as IVF have flourished (Kahn, 2000).

Alongside the drive for quantity and reproduction, Jewish-Israeli society has also emphasized quality and selection. Historically, these two emphases were combined as part of the Zionist project to build a "new people for a new land," and to replace diasporic weakness and 'effeminate submissiveness' with masculine vigor and 'Judaism with muscles' (Max Nordau's term, coined in 1898; see also Weiss, 2002; Falk, 1998). The drive for "reproducing Jews" (quantity) was thus accompanied by an emphasis on the health of progeny (quality). Since the last decade, advances in genetic technologies alongside the opening up of the health market for competition have prompted an increasingly growing use of genetic tests in Israel. Subsidized IVF now exists in Israel side-by-side with state-paid genetic screening. The growing use among secular Israelis of prenatal genetic diagnosis, combined with a continuing decrease in their average family size, probably also reflect individualistic concerns.

Prenatal diagnosis is now a widespread phenomenon in Israel. Compared to other industrialized countries, Israel has one of the broadest prenatal diagnostic programs to detect fetal anomalies. The National Health Law of 1994 defines the prenatal genetic tests to be paid for by the state. It includes three categories: amniocentesis for women who are aged 35 years or older at the beginning of the pregnancy (as part of a State subsidized program for the prenatal detection of Down syndrome), carrier detection screening for Tay-Sachs (in the past recommended only for Ashkenazi Jews but now for all Jews) and thalassemia for high risk groups (Zlotogora & Leventhal, 2000). The tests offered by the Health Management Organizations (HMOs) include a combined test of the levels of alpha-fetoprotein, human chorionic gonadotropin hormone and estriol in maternal serum (the triple test, subsidized at $15 by the HMOs for all women irrespective of age), amniocentesis and first level fetal ultrasound (Sher et al., 2003).

In addition, there are many prenatal genetic tests (that cost about $100 a test) that individuals may choose to perform privately. The number of prenatal genetic tests is constantly increasing, and so is the proportion of women using them. Out of 377 Jewish Israeli women who were surveyed in maternity wards in 2002 (Sher et al., 2003), 61% performed the triple test (as opposed to only 7% of the ultrareligious women), and 94% of the secular women older than 35 years performed amniocentesis (in contrast to 36% of the religious, and none of the ultrareligious). Being secular, having a higher income and a supplementary medical insurance, fewer children, and being of Ashkenazi origin were found to be significant factors in determining performance of genetic tests (Sher et al., 2003). A very high number of non-recommended amniocenteses are performed in Israel (for a Down syndrome risk that is lower than 1:380). According to geneticists, this is most likely due to the social emphasis placed in Israeli society on general health, and especially on the health of children (Shohat et al., 2003). In sum, the popularity of prenatal genetic testing among secular Israelis is influenced by various factors such as individual concerns, the availability of state-subsidized prenatal diagnosis, and a medical establishment that, generally speaking, legitimizes directivity (Shuval & Anson, 2000) and even eugenics (Wertz, 1998; Weiss, 2002).

While prenatal genetic testing is popular among secular Israeli individuals, premarital genetic testing is collectively practiced by the ultra-orthodox Jews. The Dor Yeshorim program mentioned before is supported by both the Israeli State and many Israeli geneticists (Sagi, 1998). This context may explain, in part at least, the drive to translate genetic lab findings into a culturally-tailored counseling scheme for "carrier matching" offered to the Bedouin community. Careful analysis is needed, however, to explore the motives of health professionals as well as community members, and the negotiated meanings of genetic counseling that were shaped within the complex interplay of tradition, ethnicity, medicalization, and the politics of reproduction.

Chapter 2

The Setting

This study sets out to describe and analyze a model for cross-cultural education and community engagement in the context of genetic counseling. The analysis focuses on an ethnographic setting where genetic tests are in the process of being offered to a particular at-risk community. This is currently the situation in the Negev Bedouin population of southern Israel. I intend to focus on this population for the purposes of the study.

At the time of the study, ten Mother and Child Health (MCH) clinics served the Bedouin living in planned towns, while the rest of the Bedouin population living in encampments (about 60,000 people) had to travel to receive this service. Staff shortages in these clinics were severe. MCH clinic nurses (most of them Jewish) made all referrals to genetic counseling and prenatal tests. All pregnant women were offered a maternal serum triple test, which entailed a fee of 15 USD for health-insured women. Second-trimester ultrasound covered by health insurance was recommended at 18–22 weeks of gestation to all pregnant women. Amniocentesis was offered free of charge by MCH clinic nurses to all women over 35 years of age at the time of conception. Amniocentesis was also offered free of charge for those at risk higher than 1:380 for Down syndrome and other genetic disorders as indicated by the triple test. CVS was rarely offered during the study period.

In 2000, 90% of the pupils in the school for the hearing-impaired, located in Beer-Sheva, were Bedouin. There was no school for the hearing-impaired in any of the Bedouin towns. Although the vast majority at school, Bedouin pupils had to study in Hebrew since none of the (Jewish) teachers spoke or signed Arabic. This situation has recently led Bedouin parents to move their hearing-impaired children to a local school in one of the Bedouin towns. The hearing impairment diagnostic kit used by the Ministry of Education was written and standardized for Hebrew speakers and was not adapted to Arabic. Cochlear implants are not provided in the local medical center in Beer-Sheva. The implant requires complementary speech therapy in Arabic, which is not available in any event due to the lack of an Arabic-speaking trained speech therapist in the Negev area. All these drawbacks present major obstacles for the provision of health services. For many Bedouin and Israelis, these drawbacks represent discrimination in resource allocation.

The Bedouin as a Target Community for Genetic Counseling

A hierarchical order is maintained within Bedouin society and family, preserving the dominance of male over female and older over younger (Marks, 1974). The high prevalence of recessive genetic diseases among the Bedouin is the result of frequent consanguineous marriages and a low rate of prenatal testing. Bedouin consanguinity traditionally involves marriage between patrilateral parallel first cousins, which is characteristic of Arab Muslim societies (Davis, 1977). Marks (1974) explained cousin marriage among the Bedouin as a factor contributing to the clustering of men into 'co-liable groups.' The first right of a Bedouin man to marry his cousin (*awlād 'amm*) is functional in sustaining clan (*khamule*) borders and implies respect for one's family. Patrilateral parallel cousin marriage is not a rule, but an advisable way to conduct affairs in the Bedouin community (Kressel, 1992:120).

When cousin marriage is not feasible, alternate choices (in descending order) consist of more distant paternal kin, agnates and group members in general, and finally strangers (Kressel, 1980). These categories can be imagined as concentric circles, which grow in circumference until reaching the outermost circle of group affiliation, with cousin marriage in the innermost circle. The Bedouin clan is therefore largely endogamous. Social identities and interactions among the Bedouin are by and large determined by this system of concentric circles, which constitute the practical expression of collectivism.

There are three major categories in the Bedouin social structure: *'abid*, *fellahin*, and clans (see also Jakubovska, 1990; Kressel, 1980; Marks, 1974). Sudanese slavery, once practiced by the Bedouin, was forbidden by the Ottoman authorities at the turn of the 20th century, yet the 'slaves' (*'abid*) remained a distinct social category. The peasants (*fellahin*), who no longer practice agriculture, similarly constitute a distinct social group. These two groups have not been incorporated into the land-owning lineage structure of tribes, which are themselves divided according to social ranking. Despite long years of co-residence and cultural homogeneity, the frequency of inter-group marriage among these categories is relatively low (less than 10% in Kressel, 1980). Inter-group marriages are also negotiated in order to reflect rank hierarchy. As Kressel (1980) showed, dominant families and clans give out fewer brides in exogamy relative to the larger number of "stranger" or agnatic outsider (*gharība*) brides taken for their sons.

Gender segregation among the Bedouin is widespread. The social status of women is based largely on marriage and rearing children. A good wife and mother is expected not to be absent from her husband's home except for everyday chores and to be self-sacrificing for the sake of the family (Mass and Al-Krenawi, 1994). Ubiquitous forms of family and community surveillance and control maintain women's sexual integrity. Dating is prohibited, romantic love is rare, and most marriages are arranged by family members in order to further promote inter- and intra-family ties. In Bedouin society, it is common for women caught in pre- or extramarital affairs to be killed by an immediate family member in order to preserve the family honor, and to erase the shame that was perceived to have been brought to the family (Mernissi, 1991). Ritual female genital surgery (RFGS) is still practiced among several Bedouin tribes. Much like patrilateral parallel cousin marriage, RFGS is not a religious commandment of the Quran or any other religion but a widespread and strongly held custom. The age for RFGS is 12 to 17 years, after menarche but before marriage. The ritual is decided on and performed by women alone. Bedouin women who were interviewed on this practice by a social worker (Asali et al., 1995) said that after RFGS women are cleaner (The Arabic word for RFGS is *tohor*—purification). A recent press campaign in Israel assumed that the practice involves clitoridectomy, is motivated by male desire to dominate and humiliate women, and that the practice should be vigorously outlawed. Many in the Bedouin community, including Bedouin gynecologists working in the local Israeli medical center, argue that the ritual involves mostly female attitudes and always female perpetuators, and is today in Israel a non-mutilative operation akin to male circumcision (Asali et al., 1995).

Bedouin men usually work in semi-professional blue-collar jobs. There is a very high rate of unemployment, which is estimated at 25 percent in the towns. In the "unrecognized" villages the rate is probably much higher (Abu-Rabi'a, 2000). The average size of a Bedouin family is 9.5. Consanguinity is estimated at 50–60%, about half of which is patrilateral parallel cousin marriage (Weitzman et al., 2000). Polygyny is also common (an estimated 17–20% of the married women are not first wives). This population is characterized by a high fertility rate—estimated at 40–60 births annually per 1000 women at child bearing age, with a total fertility rate of married Bedouin women being about 4.75 in towns and 6.85 in rural villages (Gilbar 1997; Borkan et al., 2000). Low socioeconomic status, and a high rate of illiteracy, especially among women, are characteristic of this population (Meir, 1997).

Almost all Bedouin women attend the local medical center for childbirth. Bedouin women receive Maternal and Child Health (MCH) care at clinics run by the Ministry of Health, where prenatal examinations and child health surveillance are performed. Utilization of this service is quite high (about 89%; see Weitzman et al., 2000). Infant mortality among the Bedouin is about 13.1 per 1000 live births (about 3.5 times higher than the Jewish population). It has been estimated that in the last decade, about 50% of infant deaths in Bedouin families were due to congenital defects and hereditary diseases. At the same time, less than 10 percent of eligible Bedouin women used amniocentesis, compared to about 50 percent of Jewish women in the area (Davidov et al., 1994). One of the obvious reasons for not being tested is the Muslim objection to abortion. As a result of genetic studies that began around 1992, over 10 recessive disease genes have been mapped in the Negev Bedouin population (Sheffield et al., 1994; Carmi et al., 1994, 1995; Walder et al., 1997). The combination of frequent consanguinity and a religious ban on abortion, which made prenatal counseling largely irrelevant, motivated counselors to offer the community the use of premarital carrier matching.

The subpopulations that were targeted for this study are two Bedouin communities. The first community comprises about 3,000 individuals (additional identifying details or maps are not presented in order to shelter the anonymity of the researchees) living in a shantytown. Congenital hearing loss or "non-syndromic recessive deafness" (NSRD) has been diagnosed in over 100 clan members in the last three generations (Scott et al., 1998). The actual prevalence is evidently higher since many of the older clan members did not undergo any screening or diagnosis procedure. Part of this population is also affected by arthrogryposis, a congenital condition characterized by multiple joint contractures, frequently accompanied by muscle weakness. A genetic test for arthrogryposis will hopefully soon be offered to the community (personal interview with the Head of the Genetics Institute. This population is characterized by low socioeconomic and educational levels, high fertility rates, low availability and/or poor utilization of prenatal services, and religious restrictions on pregnancy termination. Detailed sociodemographic and epidemiological data regarding this population are presented in chapter four. Genetic estimates suggest that about 20–25% of the study population are carriers of the NSRD mutation. The second subpopulation, which is affected by a high incidence of thalassemia, lives in a Bedouin town. This group (clan or *khamule)* comprises about 600 people characterized by a relatively high socioeconomic status (as compared to the first group) and by higher levels of education. Consanguinity was also prevalent in this group.

The Background of the Genetics Program

The impetus for the program came from a medical geneticist working in the local hospital, who told me (personal interview) that she saw the program as "bringing back to community members the results of genetic research in which they were originally the subjects." About ten years before this program was launched, the same geneticist had initiated an educational campaign against inter-marriage in an extended Bedouin family congenitally afflicted with a metabolic disease causing death at around four weeks of age. This "well intended but naive intervention" (Carmi et al., 1998: 393) resulted in family disputes between young men who out-married and their parents. In addition, young and healthy unmarried women from that family were stigmatized and were consequently inter-married as second and third wives within the clan.[1] The current rationale for the program should be understood against the backdrop of this early and unsuccessful attempt.

A community-based program to reduce the incidence of congenital anomalies and hereditary diseases among the Negev Bedouin has been officially funded by the Israeli Ministry of Health since 1994, through the Committee on Reducing Infant Mortality. The program and its preliminary study were conducted by the Regional office of the Ministry of Health, the Department of Epidemiology and Health Services Evaluation at the Faculty of Health Sciences at Ben-Gurion University, and the Genetics Institute at the Soroka Medical Center. It began implementation in the largest Bedouin town in the Negev (population 30,000), and was later extended to other Bedouin towns and villages. The main goals of the program were genetic education informing the local population about the risks inherent in consanguinity, as well as improved accessibility to genetic counseling services which prior to the project had been provided only in Beer-Sheva, the Negev's largest (Jewish) city. Local women from the community specially trained by the research team to serve as peer instructors performed educational activities. These community-outreach instructors worked in the Maternal and Child Health (MCH) clinics where almost all Bedouin women visit either for prenatal care or for follow-up and immunizations. With the aid of a specially designed brochure, the process, timing and purpose of genetic tests were explained. Women were encouraged to use genetic counseling and prenatal diagnostic tests and to initiate prenatal care early in their next pregnancy. To improve accessibility, a community-based referral service was introduced. A local Bedouin person with medical

---

1. Being a second or third wife usually means an inferior status in relation to the first wife.

education was specially trained to interview women belonging to high risk families, where genetic diseases amenable for prenatal diagnosis existed. These women were referred from the local four MCH clinics in order to assess their level of risk and to further refer them for diagnostic tests in the Genetics Institute. Additional educational activities included a region-wide workshop on consanguinity for health professionals and social workers serving the Bedouin population, an update course for nurses working in clinics that serve Bedouin communities on prental diagnostic tests available for the Bedouin population, and a special curriculum for Bedouin high school students to teach human genetics. Teachers who work with the Bedouin were offered a special workshop on teaching genetics.

The intervention program departed from the conventional clinical-diagnostic model; many of its activities took place not in a health care facility in response to some medical complaint, but rather in the community and at school. Unlike other programs in the west, which are usually administered to heterogeneous populations on a federal or national basis, this program was designed for a homogeneous ethnic minority through a participatory process involving community members as outreach assistants.

The experimental program for carrier matching, which is the focus of this study, was therefore only one activity (and certainly not the central one) of the entire regional project that was initiated and funded by the Ministry of Health to reduce the incidence of hereditary diseases. NSRD tests, for example, were paid for by funds available to the Genetics Institute, and not by the Ministry of Health. The experimental program for carrier matching reflected, in the eyes of professionals, a cultural adaptation to Bedouin norms. Because abortion was not an accepted option, the program focused on pre-marital (rather than prenatal) counseling. In order to reduce the risk of stigmatization (especially for women), carrier status was not individually disclosed. Rather, it was decided with the targeted community to employ a system of carrier matching which can be termed "integrative disclosure." In this system, potential partners are told if they are genetically "compatible" or not ("incompatibility" meaning the two partners being carriers, thus having a 25% risk at each pregnancy of having an affected child). If neither or just one of the two partners is a carrier, they are told that they are genetically "compatible." At the same time, an alternative option is provided where personal tests can be taken (for the standard cost of about US$ 100),[2] and results are dis-

2. The Israeli national health insurance law defines various services which are provided for free. The above-mentioned genetic test is currently not part of these state-subsidized services and therefore has to be paid for by those using it.

closed through regular procedures of genetic counseling. Premarital screening was offered for congenital hearing loss (NSRD) and later thalassemia was planned to be included.

A public meeting, in which a group of health professionals presented and discussed the idea of the program with community members for the first time, took place in June 1998. Publicizing the meeting presented a problem. Since there was no mail service in the ("unrecognized") village, invitations could not be mailed. Neither was there any directory of telephone numbers. Notifications about the public meeting were hand-delivered from home to home by two community-outreach Arabic speaking individuals (a local Bedouin man and an Arab-Israeli woman), who also gave more information about the purpose of the meeting. The meeting took place at the local school, considered to be a well-known, neutral and central place. About 50 Bedouin men of various ages attended the meeting. Bedouin women are customarily prohibited from attending public meetings together with men. Translation into sign language was not provided. Following the presentation by health professionals (in Hebrew and Arabic), one of the Bedouin men asked: "What about a cure?" to which one of the doctors answered: "There is no medication. We can avoid the birth of sick people by raising the community's awareness and preparing to participate in the program."[3] Another doctor repeated the explanation about the recessive nature of the disease, and stressed the relevance of the system employed by *Dor Yeshorim,* the importance of confidentiality and informed consent, the positive attitude of Islam towards science, and the importance of home instruction. When he was finished, one of the Bedouin said: "We are ready to begin as soon as possible." Additional questions from the floor soon followed: "Do you provide an answer on the spot?" "What about other diseases, do you have a test for them?" "It is difficult to bring my daughter to the Genetics Institute, what do you suggest? "Does all the family need to come?" "What ages will be tested?" "What about the problem of marriage?" The professional answers to these questions will be explicated below in a section dealing with the design of the program. However, many of the questions needed to be negotiated on a practical basis during the implementation of the program. These questions therefore set the scene for the unfolding of the program.

3. Description of the meeting is based on interviews conducted with individuals who attended it.

The Social Construction of Congenital Hearing Loss among the Bedouin

Genetic tests for NSRD were offered since in public meetings many Bedouin stated that hearing impairment was a disadvantage. Many of the men present at the meetings said that while marrying out of the tribe was difficult, it would be a good idea to use carrier matching in order to prevent the birth of deaf children. Those who came to the meetings, however, were often a-priori more in favor of the idea of genetic counseling. The voices of those against it were under-represented in these meetings.

In interviews I conducted, the picture was more complex. The first reply of many Bedouin was that "deafness is from *Allah* (God)." When asked what they thought about the life of the hearing-impaired, some Bedouin respondents said that "deaf people are likely to have difficulties finding and keeping a job," and that "deaf women are likely to be married as second, rather than first wives." These respondents considered hearing impairment to be a handicap and a disadvantage. However, other Bedouin respondents also said, in regard to the marriage prospects of the hearing impaired, that it is customary to match older women with deaf men. In their view, it was better for these older (and non-deaf) women to get married with a deaf man than not to be married at all. Still other Bedouin respondents claimed that "deafness is not a burden," and that "deaf children grow up capable of doing everything, just like hearing people." One respondent (the father of two hearing-impaired boys) even claimed that "deaf children are better since they are more quiet and easier to take care of at home." Another Bedouin respondent (the mother of two hearing-impaired children, a boy and a girl) said: "deaf people may have difficulties getting and keeping a job, but even if they don't have a job, they can get money from social security, so this is not really a problem."

Two opposing paradigms of cultural interaction can be found in the literature regarding hearing-impaired individuals. The first category, cultural assimilation, is best represented by Nora Groce's (1985) intriguing study on Martha's Vineyard—an inbred island community not far from Boston, MA, with a high incidence of hereditary hearing loss, where "everyone spoke sign language" and the hearing-impaired were integrated into all facets of life. The second category, cultural differentiation, is represented by Deaf culture. Deaf culture emphasizes pride, resistance and mobilization in response to how the 'hearing world' classifies people who are hearing-impaired. Deaf people struggle to re-frame the disadvantage that results from negative attitudes of a hearing society that fails to communicate with them effectively. Deaf culture, then, celebrates the difference of hearing loss rather than looking for ways to assimilate into the 'hearing world.' Different sign languages and Deaf social clubs have emerged as predominant symbols and means for the construction of a positive social identity and cohesion (Ladd, 1990,1991; Atkin et al., 2002).

The Bedouin community is located in between these two categories, closer to the assimilation pole than to differentiation. Deaf culture is currently not available, even as an idea, as an option for resistance and mobilization. This is due both to economic hardships and to the dominance of traditional norms. The premises of Deaf culture, hinging on liberal individualism and cultural diversity, appear to be too foreign for Bedouin culture. Indeed, studies in the UK and the US have shown that Deaf culture is practiced mainly by white, professional, middle class individuals, and is criticized by minority ethnic deaf people and their families for not responding to ethnic and religious diversity (Ahmad et al., 1998).

While Deaf culture is not an option, assimilation is something that can be aspired for but is not often achieved. More and more Bedouin increasingly consider deafness to be a handicap and a disadvantage, even if not a stigma. It is possible that a few decades ago hearing-impaired individuals were considered an integral part of the community and assimilated into the 'hearing world.' Echoes of this recent era are heard, for example, in the following interview excerpt:

> "My father was deaf but that didn't bother our family. His work was to take care of the family's herd of sheep. I have seven brothers and sisters, some of them deaf and some can hear. He treated all of us in the same way. My mother was not deaf, and I do not remember her discussing father's deafness in a negative manner" (interview with a Bedouin woman, age 22).

Additional indications of assimilation are the existence, in those parts of the clan where hearing loss was prevalent, of a relatively common use of a local sign language by hearing and deaf people alike (Kisch, 2000). However, even in a situation where hearing people understand sign language, the hearing-impaired are still disadvantaged since they require translation of spoken language. In addition, hearing loss is not subjected to treatment by local healers (perhaps because they cannot offer any remedy) and there is no ethnographic evidence for any moral meaning attached to it (Kisch, 2000: 201).

The process of modernization accentuated the disadvantages of hearing loss for men and consequently for women, too. It is relatively more difficult for hearing-impaired Bedouin men to be hired for many types of manual labor (driving, construction and shop floor work, for example), which are usually supervised by Jewish-Israelis and in which many hearing Bedouin work. Professional and white-collar occupations are largely beyond the reach of hearing-impaired Bedouin due to lack of proper education and support. The "marriage value" (to use a Bedouin expression) of deaf women is lower, and they are usually married as second wives. These norms are a reflection of the traditional, patriarchal Bedouin worldview. Indeed, one of the goals of the experimental program for carrier matching was to reduce the stigmatization of hearing-impaired individuals (particularly women) through genetics education and the practice of confidential carrier matching (entitled "integrative disclosure"). In practice, it should be noted, the genetics program itself could inadvertently contribute to stigmatization due to the medicalization of hearing loss.

A recently-established support network for Bedouin parents of children with disabilities, currently active in the city of Beer-Sheva and the Bedouin town of Tel-Sheva, comprised at the time of the study about 80 members and included a strong group of parents of deaf children. Members were generally of a relatively high socio-economic status, with occupations such as schoolteachers, engineers, lawyers, and other urban professionals. The network was organized by *Shatil*, a non-governmental Israeli organization which coaches third-sector and voluntary associations at the grass-root level. A *Shatil* worker, who was also a Bedouin, coordinated the meetings. There were no women in the group. According to the coordinator (personal communication, February 4, 2000), parents of deaf children had a strong presence in the group because, on the one hand, they did not see deafness as a stigma, while on the other hand they had a lot of problems to share. While this group could demonstrate a possible venue of change for Bedouin society, it should be stressed that the socio-economic characteristics of its participants were hardly representative.

In contrast to hearing loss, thalassemia is a severe, life-threatening disease that requires life-long treatment (blood transfusion at 4–6 weekly intervals). Treatment is provided only in the medical center in the city of Beer-Sheva. An affected child will die without transfusion and iron-chelating drugs. However necessary, the treatment is also aggressive, demanding and burdensome (see also Modell and Berdoukas, 1984). Bone marrow transplantation, notwithstanding its possible complications, offers a potential cure and is particularly relevant to populations like the Bedouin that prefer patrilateral parallel cousin marriage and have large families, as both these factors increase the chance of finding a compatible donor. In interviews with community members, there was a consensus that thalassemia was a severe disease that is better avoided. During home interviews conducted with more than half the targeted clan where thalassemia was prevalent, all the Bedouin respondents confirmed their wish to receive genetic counseling for thalassemia. As the thalassemia project is still in its early stages this data should be regarded as preliminary.

The Design of the Program for Carrier Matching

The program's rationale followed that of *Dor Yeshorim,* the successful genetics program developed more than a decade ago by the global orthodox Ashkenazi-Jewish community. The professionals behind the Bedouin program were quite familiar with *Dor Yeshorim* and referred to it as their model. According to their explanation, the Jewish and Bedouin communities shared—despite considerable differences—two normative similarities: (a) Marriages are often pre-arranged, and consanguinity is the main reason for a high prevalence of genetic diseases, and (b) there is a religious ban on abortion.[4] Several basic differences existed in the application of genetic counseling in the two communities. Unlike *Dor Yeshorim,* the Bedouin were offered only the test for NSRD (a relatively non-severe condition). The test for thalassemia was offered to a different Bedouin sub-population where the condition was prevalent. Unlike the Orthodox Jewish community, the Bedouin do not have a strong central leadership, religious or otherwise, and the program for carrier matching therefore had to be offered to community members through public education, home instructions and public meetings. In addition, the Bedouin's uptake of medical services in general is known to be low because of problems of accessibility as well as cultural differences.

The NSRD program for carrier matching unfolded along four major stages: community involvement, community instruction, blood drawing, and genetic counseling. The thalassemia program was, in principle, designed to follow the same stages. Both targeted populations agreed to participate in a program comprising at-home instructions, genetic testing, and genetic counseling. In each community, the implementation of the program ideally comprised the following six essential steps:

1. Population survey to assess gene frequency
2. Preliminary public meeting with community members, informing them about the following steps of the program, and receiving their consent to participate

4. For discussion on Muslim attitudes toward abortion, see Rispler-Chaim (1999) and Rogers (1999).

3. Home instructions that include the following components:
- Collection of basic personal data (names, family pedigree, etc.)
- Instruction regarding the relevant disease/congenital disorder, genetic risk and etiology, and relation to consanguinity. All the services and treatments available in regard to the disease/condition, as well as the costs and difficulties, were to be explained in this stage. In addition, the instructor introduced the various options of premarital testing (individual, stepwise and carrier-matching). Members of the community, who were recruited and trained for that purpose, provided this instruction in Arabic. The instruction was interactive and made use of flip charts, posters and other graphic materials.
- Group discussions on the question "which counseling format is most suitable for your family." The discussion was moderated by the instructor, who wrote down the attitudes and arguments of family members in their own words. This "natural group interview" provided a local equivalent to the more contrived focus group used in attitude research (Beckerleg et al., 1997).
4. Second meeting with the family about 1–2 weeks following instruction in order to ascertain what decision they had reached and whether it represented a consensus or not.
5. Definition of preferred patterns of testing and counseling, coordination of location and dates for testing and counseling.
6. Monitoring and follow-up on utilization

The genetics education, instruction, and counseling were similar for all families. Obviously, there were different emphases in the contents of instruction, reflecting the diseases (NSRD/thalassemia) prevalent in the communities. For this reason, the data are presented in a general way, except for specific places in which I analyze the impact of the severity of the disease on emerging patterns of attitudes and utilization.

Methodological Considerations

Typically, discussions of methodology are presented in either a qualitative or a quantitative category because the two paradigms have been assumed to be polar opposites. This study, in contrast, combines both methods. This follows the contention that quantitative and qualitative methodologies can be viewed on a continuum and that each approach adds to the body of knowledge by building on the information derived from the other approach (see also Newman and Benz, 1998). For example, qualitative methodology can be suitably used to elicit themes and concepts that reflect Bedouin as well as professional attitudes towards cross-cultural genetics education. These inductive concepts can then be used in a questionnaire in order to quantitatively test their interpretation by various groups in the population. In a similar manner, statistical results of a questionnaire can be further explained by using open interviews and focus groups.

The juxtaposition of in-depth interviews and statistical analysis can be baffling to some readers, who are more accustomed to the professional separation of these sources of data. I believe there is much to be gained from such a combination of "the best of both worlds." Quantitative-qualitative feedback loops can actually enhance the validity of the study. Such combined research builds on and extends the methodological principle of triangulation (obtaining a variety of data sources in order to have a complete perception of the phenomenon) advocated by Denzin (1978), for example. While not purporting to reconcile the philosophical differences between positivistic and naturalistic stances, my pragmatic argument is that one needs to identify qualitative and/or quantitative research according to the type of question being asked and the type of data being collected.

The analysis focuses on four general sources of data: interviews, questionnaires, observations, and textual analysis. Data were collected using these methods in both sub-populations that were targeted for the study, namely the community that was at risk for NSRD and the community that was at risk for thalassemia.

1. Interviews. Several rounds of interviews were conducted by the research assistants and me since 1999 with the following groups of people: (a) six genetic counselors (including community-outreach assistants) as well as five health professionals involved in the program; (b) six Bedouin couples and six Bedouin individuals who came for genetic counseling; and (c) 38 adult members of nine families, chosen as a representative sample of different categories of utilization/compliance. This sample was also stratified by level of known genetic risk, age and gender. In addition, interviews were conducted with health professionals and genetic counselors from Tel-Aviv and Jerusalem, who were involved in genetic screening for Arab-Israelis and Orthodox Ashkenazi Jews. The Bedouin community-outreach liaison person had many talks about genetic testing, consanguinity and carrier matching with various community members. We discussed these talks in regular meetings held every week.

I observed several of the counseling sessions with the consent of the counselees. All counselees were interviewed separately a few days after the session and asked about their motivations and expectations. The counselor who conducted the session was interviewed the next day, and counselees were interviewed for a second time a few weeks later to follow up on their decision-making process. All these interviews were semi-structured, and lasted from one to three hours. They were held in various places, from the home to the hospital, according to the respondents' convenience. Interviews were conducted mostly in Hebrew, a language in which most Bedouin men are quite fluent. Where needed, Arabic was used and translated. Many of the respondents perceived me, a Jewish researcher working at the local university, as a representative of the genetics program. I therefore explained that the interview was not part of the actual program and that its goal was to hear people's genuine opinions, including their criticism, so that the program could be improved. The fact that such criticism was voiced and that the research assistants and myself encountered a plurality of opinions was a positive indication.

In order to understand the attitudes of Bedouin women in regard to the program, a female researcher conducted interviews in Arabic with 28 women. Almost all these interviews were conducted in the respondents' home, late in the morning, while the house was relatively quiet. The group's composition represented all the important categories of the study population. 24 women received instruction while four were married to men who refused to receive instruction. 14 were married, 10 of them being the first wife and 4 the second wife. Eight were unmarried women who had already been genetically tested but have not yet come for counseling. Three women in this group participated in counseling for carrier matching.

Questions used in the interviews with Bedouin men and women included perceptions of genetic testing and of cousin marriage, specifically in terms of genetic risk, social goals, paternal authority, and romantic love. These questions were asked by the research assistants and me in an open-ended manner (without offering specific options for responses, so as to let respondents speak their minds in their own words). While the interview was structured around these standard questions, open discussions also developed around particular questions. A brief summary of the research was presented to each interviewee prior to the interview. All participants had the right to refrain from answering any question and could also withdraw from the interview at any time. The transcribed interviews were analyzed reaching agreement between the researchers on categorization of attitudes related to each question. Disagreements were resolved by discussion.

Information collected through the interviews included the following main categories:

I. Basic demographic data. Number of children, age, gender, marital status, health, and detailed information about familial proximity to affected individuals. Data was stored in a "family tree" software program.

II. Factors associated with participation, acceptance and use of test results. Interviews were designed to assess (a) Health belief components hypothesized to affect program-related attitudes and behaviors; (b) Family-related, ethnic, traditional, and cultural factors hypothesized to affect decisions about the actual use of genetic test results.

III. Preferences regarding the use of test results for making decisions about marriage and /or family planning. Attitudes towards all possible counseling options were thematized and analyzed. This included carrier matching, individual and stepwise disclosure, with or without an intention to use prenatal diagnosis (CVS or amniocentesis). Socio-demographic data and actual attitudes were tested for statistical correlations.

Interviews were also conducted with all the program staff (mainly the genetic counselors) and other professionals involved. These interviews focused on the attitudes of counselors and health professionals towards the program and its dynamics.

2. *Observations.* In addition to the counseling sessions that were observed with the consent of counselees, at-home instruction sessions provided another source of observational material. A total of about 65 instruction sessions were conducted since 2000, of which 10 were analyzed in detail. In addition, observations were conducted in training sessions for instructors and in the program's staff meetings, as well as in public meetings with the community. Observations were thematically analyzed with regard to attitudes in practice, and compared to the interviews.

3. *Texts.* Textual analysis included educational materials used in the instruction sessions (English, Hebrew and Arabic versions), forms and reports, and short summaries of counseling sessions with community members, which were prepared by the genetic counselors.

All this information was brought together using several categories. Bedouin attitudes were thematized according to three basic categories that emanated from the interviews and observations: compliance, utilization, and rejection. These categories were further analyzed so as to compare formal attitudes expressed in public settings and informal attitudes expressed in everyday life. The attitudes of professionals were also thematized according to their position in regard to the ethical dilemmas that characterized the program.

In addition, during 2001 meetings were conducted with five groups of Bedouin pupils and seven groups of their teachers. These groups represented Bedouin schools in cities as well as in "unrecognized" areas that serve shantytowns and encampments. The five groups of pupils (n=40) represented five different schools, which all had the same curriculum in human genetics. The seven groups of teachers (n=61) were recruited from the same schools as well as from other schools in the area. A questionnaire concerning knowledge of genetics and attitudes towards genetic testing and counseling was administered to the pupils and teachers. During 2002, six more meetings with a total of 81 participants were conducted in Bedouin schools with the educational film 'Āysha' serving as a focal point for discussion. To evaluate the effects of cultural norms, ethnicity and counseling style on the interpretation of nondirectiveness, another questionnaire was administered to 281 Jewish and 133 Bedouin respondents.

Access to information was gained through my role in the program for carrier matching, which was initially one of evaluation. My initial task was to evaluate the Bedouin response to genetic testing. Interviews conducted with the Bedouin were analyzed according to the Health Belief Model (Kirscht, 1988). This research tested hypotheses on the influence of such parameters as education, susceptibility, social status, religiosity, and perceived marriage prospects on program utilization. Later I also became, for a brief period of time, Chair of the program's ethics committee. While the evaluative part of the study had a positivistic emphasis on quantitative results and hypothesis-testing within pre-conceived models, the present work represents a post-positivistic, interpretive emphasis, which to my mind is no less important for purposes of analysis as well as evaluation. Symbolic interactionism was not a declared part of the evaluative research from its outset, but it nevertheless guided my data collection and analysis. An important reason for entering the program and studying genetic counseling was my realization, from the outset, that it was a case of glocalization (Raz, 1999), where symbolic interactionism could make a theoretical and analytical difference.

Researching and Intervening: Ethnographic Reflection

This study involved theory and practice, research and implementation, observation as well as intervention. This combination has its unique quandaries. Before discussing them, I would like to present in detail one of the earlier interviews I conducted in the Bedouin community. I met Hussein (pseudonym) and his family in their house. Hussein was a member of the Bedouin community where NSRD screening has been under implementation. The community liaison told me before the interview that Hussein was unemployed, did not attend instruction, and had a wife and children who were not tested in the program. I was also told that Hussein recently engaged his daughter to a clan member after this man took an individual test and was not found to be a carrier. I parked the car near two small houses, one of them still under construction. As the research assistant, Hussein and myself entered the guestroom, he introduced us to his wife and three of his young children. One of the boys started to cry. Hussein told him: "don't worry my son, they are not doctors." The following exchange was transcribed, excerpted and translated from the interview, which took about an hour.

Hussein: "I haven't worked for some time. I have had this disease [specific details are not given in order to shelter the anonymyty of the respondent] since about six years ago. Some people here will tell you I'm not part of the tribe at all, because I used to live in another city for long time, 15, maybe 16 years. After I stopped being employed, I became sick."

I: "Is there any particular reason why you didn't attend the instruction?"

Hussein: "We didn't do it, we were visiting family. Personally we didn't do it. The instructors came to our neighbors, and my wife heard it. I didn't hear it, but I was involved in it a lot."

I: "What do you think about carrier matching for inherited deafness?"

Hussein: "There are more severe diseases, that's for sure. There are worse things...." At this point Hussein stopped, turned to the research assistant, a young woman who engaged his wife in conversation, and interrupted them by asking: "What did you ask her?"

Assistant: "I asked about the tests your son-in-law did."

Hussein: "No, you have to see.... They said that if one carries the gene, then it's enough that one does the test. So he did it. It's not something.... He's a person, how to say, he's not primitive or anything, so he didn't take offense, so he did it."

Assistant: "Did you ask him to?"

Hussein: "No, I didn't ask, I said to him, I told him it would be good for both of them. Although I know that we, my family, we don't have that gene. My family's branch does not have any case of deafness. Not my brothers, not my father, not my cousins."

I: "So he took the test on his own? And what happened then?"

Hussein: "Well, he got an answer that he wasn't a carrier."

I: "What would have happened if he got another answer?"

Hussein: "Look, if I'm not a carrier and my wife is not a carrier, then it's clear that our children are not carriers, right?"

I: "That's right. But you didn't take the test."

Hussein (determined): "I am sure we're not carriers, my wife and I. I look at the family, and I think that today, in this clan, we're definitely the family with the least risk."

I: "Why do you think we give answers only to couples, not to individuals?"
Hussein: "But it's confidential. I can do the test with money, right?" [Meaning paying for an individual test]
I: "Yes."
Hussein: "I can do it with money and know what the situation is. Why don't you do it like this for everyone?"
I: "We're afraid that if someone gets an answer that she's a carrier, it would make it difficult for her to marry."
Hussein: "See, I'm looking at the full half of the glass, like they say.... If I could know right away.... According to the test, I would know for sure. I could know tomorrow. The children don't need to know. I did it like that because Fā'iza [pseudonym for his engaged daughter] was too young then. If she was 20 years old, I wouldn't mind her taking the test."
I: "But you preferred that the intended groom do the test first."
Hussein: "I could do it without the groom. Once she's all right, I don't care about the groom. In terms of matching."
I: "Please excuse me, I didn't understand why you said she was too young. Age is not supposed to matter in terms of taking the test."
Hussein: "Not in terms of.... But in terms of doing it, why do I need the whole story, I am not going to give myself and her that headache."
I: "So you mean you didn't tell her?"
Hussein (very softly): "No, no, why give her such a headache? I say it's better like this. We're more relaxed like this."

At this point the research assistant and Hussein's wife began to talk about Fā'iza, what she was doing and where she lived. Hussein began to cough and said that he felt a seizure was approaching and that the interview must end. We offered to give him a ride to the nearest clinic, but he refused. His final words before we left were: "You better go now.... I don't remember anything from what I said." He repeated this sentence twice.

This interview can be read in several ways. First, it illustrates the mixture of research and implementation. The context of interviewing required the appearance of neutrality on the part of the interviewer, so that respondents would feel as free as possible to share whatever attitudes they had, including negative ones. In reality, all the interviewers were identified with the program for carrier matching. This was an inevitable consequence of their positioning by the Bedouin respondents. Even if a new and unfamiliar assistant had conducted the interview, the first question of the respondent would be aimed at identifying the interviewer's role. I was quite aware of being positioned as a representative of the program since during the interview people asked me informational questions. Indeed, parts of the interviews could be seen as equivalent to instruction. I had to explain time and again that the interview was not part of the program and that its goal was to hear people's own real opinions, including their criticisms, so that the program could be improved. I even refrained, on purpose, from taking part in any public meetings of the program with the community so as not be cast as a program official. Yet I am sure that for many of the respondents, the other research assistants and I were unavoidably deemed part of the program. The interview with Hussein illustrates our strategy of neutrality in the face of Hussein's agenda. As neutral as we tried to be, Hussein's hesitations were very evident when he realized the gap between his actions and the program's rationale.

I believe Hussein's termination of the interview was due to his embarrassment for exposing the fact that he concealed his actions from his daughter. Hussein implicitly admitted in negotiating a "stepwise test" with the person who asked to marry his daughter (Fā'iza). He explained that "Fā'iza was too young to take the test." However, he said it without real confidence. His explanations about the benefit of "knowing for sure [. . . .] even tomorrow" reflected an understanding of the process of genetic counseling. Hussein also preferred to protect his daughter from potential stigmatization. It transpired that he had not thought he should involve Fā'iza in these considerations. When hearing his wife tell us about Fā'iza, he must have realized that we could also try to interview her and must have felt threatened.

Such a reading throws into relief the intricate nature of interviewing that takes place in a family context. Genetic counseling, as I noted in the introduction, involves competing perspectives of spouses, parents, or family members. Counseling should be client-led, yet the existence of multiple clients raises the question: by which client? This question is further substantiated in the interview with Hussein, which demonstrates that the perspectives of family members can indeed be in conflict. The interviewer is inevitably ensnared by such conflicts. Interviewing family members, in a group or as individuals, can raise hidden conflicts, particularly when conducted in the context of a patriarchal and status-laden population such as the Bedouin society. Such family dynamics are also part of the dialectics I termed as 'researching and intervening.'

Another reading of the interview could emphasize the notion of cultural difference. Hussein's story was evidently full of lacunas and inconsistencies. Did the groom-to-be object to the arrangement? Who actually paid for the test? Why did Hussein have to insist on a test if he truly believed, as he said, that his children were not carriers? Why did he raise Fā'iza's young age as a reason for not testing her first, when he obviously knew this was not accountable? These questions turn the interview into a detective story. While finding out the answers was a feat in itself (and one that could involve a lot of intervening), these questions could also be read on a deeper level. How much in these questions represented the existence of a cultural pattern, and how much represented Hussein's idiosyncratic actions? After all, Hussein's actions also reflected Bedouin norms, for example paternal authority. Hussein's termination of the interview showed that he resisted our questions. For him, perhaps for any Bedouin patriarch, such an interview must have appeared to be an interrogation. Some of my remarks, such as stressing that "the age does not affect the test" seem in retrospect a direct affront in Bedouin terms. Even if it were true that Hussein covered up his real intentions by using the daughter's age as an excuse, it was culturally insulting to insist on the opposite, thus implying that age was a poor excuse. During the interview, however, I (wrongly?) felt it was the most natural thing to comment on.

Interestingly, Hussein's way of ending the interview could also fit into this cultural reading. Hussein asked to finish the interview because he said he was feeling bad and was afraid that a seizure was coming on. But his final words ("I don't remember a word from what I said") could also represent denial. The use of a subjective illness experience, although quite idiosyncratic, could also reflect a Bedouin pattern. As Talal Asad (1986) argued, the rather commonly invoked model of ethnography as translation hides the fact that cultures are not like coherent languages or texts but are composed of conflicting discourses. The apparently neutral act of translation or "dialogue" is always enmeshed in power inequalities. There are "strong" and "weak" languages, and "the vast majority of ethnographies are written in strong languages" (Clifford, 1990: 58). If Hussein was feeling uncomfortable about the direction of the interview, he could (presumably) have put an end to it right there and then. He did not need an excuse to cut short the interview. Nevertheless, he preferred to end the interview by invoking what he presented as an objective condition, namely an impending seizure. If this interpretation is correct, then Hussein was using his illness as a social resource for manipulating the situation and controlling it. The next day I asked the liaison person (a Bedouin man) to call Hussein. I was told by the liaison person that Hussein said his condition improved immediately after we left.

Following the interview with Hussein, the research assistants and I decided on a few practical steps. We agreed to avoid, as much as possible, any reference to other family members. We also agreed to avoid, as much as possible, any comments that could be interpreted as critical and insulting. We also agreed that a shift in the definition of the situation was needed, since the interview was possibly interpreted by many Bedouin respondents as an extension of the program. When coordinating the interview, we presented the meeting not as an interview but rather as an opportunity for us to "see how things are with the family and what has been happening with you." To emphasize the unofficial nature of the meeting, the assistants and I decided to bring with us to the interview a small gift—usually some inexpensive toy for the children in the house.

So far I focused on the double bind of research and implementation, observation as well as intervention, in the relationships between the Bedouin respondents and me. However, the relationships between the health professionals and me were not without problems and quandaries, too. The health professionals who were involved in the experimental program for carrier matching were both colleagues and respondents. My role in the program for carrier matching was one of implementation and evaluation. In the original research proposal that provided funding for the continued implementation as well as analysis of the carrier matching program, the framing of the study was based on what I can now term as constructive reflexivity. The proposal thus stated that "the premises of the project are not taken for granted, but rather examined and questioned. The project's rationale for intervention, for example, is based on medical premises. However, whether and/or to what extent doctors' warnings are sufficient to promote a change of norms is an open question, one that will be empirically pursued in the study. [...] Clan members' attitudes derive from a combination of several discourses, medical reasoning being only one of them." In addition, the proposal offered to "examine the attitudes of both the community and the professional agents of community genetics." The methodological design thus included observations of staff meetings as well as the project's designated activities, and interviews with health professionals and genetic counselors on attitudes and decision-making processes that led to and accompanied the carrier-matching program. These observations and interviews were conducted by the principal investigator. The proposal stressed this aspect as one of its strengths, arguing that "while previous studies have focused on community attitudes, this study will also examine the professional attitudes of project staff along dimensions such as authority and empowerment, rigidity and flexibility, and nondirective neutrality and intervention." The proposal was submitted by me as the principal investigator and by two senior health professionals as co-investigators. In the same manner that I was to intervene as well as to observe, the health professionals were to be co-investigators as well as researchees. This duality formed the explicit basis for the research proposal. The double bind inherent in it, however, was made explicit only at a later stage of the research, when this book was being written.

Towards the end of the research the health professionals and I co-authored papers that presented the practical aspects of the carrier matching program and its evaluation in positivistic parameters that measure the knowledge and attitudes of community members. However, I had clarified that I also intended to write a book on the subject where I would be the single author due to the book's socio-anthropological and reflexive nature. Moreover, I gave my co-investigators an early version of the manuscript and asked for their comments. The result was a tense meeting in which the manuscript and I were criticized. I focus here on the constructive aspects of that criticism. First, my co-investigators argued that they did not anticipate that I was going to publish such a book single-handedly. Second, publishing a book was criticized as premature, given the fact that it was too early for stable patterns of utilization to emerge. My response was that in my view it was interesting and important to analyze those patterns of utilization and attitudes that have emerged during the first and formative years of the project. Third, the manuscript was criticized for containing partial information as well as data that was unethically collected, and for presenting an unjustified negative portrayal of the project's staff. This last objection highlights the unpleasant implications of the health professionals' realization of their double bind as both researchers and researchees. I explained to the health professionals, as I now explain to the readers of this book, that my interviews with them and with the project's staff were conducted as part of the research which was outlined in the proposal cited above. In the beginning of each interview I explained that this was an interview and that its purpose was to better understand the social and ethical implications of the carrier matching program. Almost all of these interviews were taped with the consent of the respondents. To shelter the anonymity of the researchees I have referred to them throughout the book as "health professionals" or "counselors," omitting all identifying details except for those which were necessary for the analysis (such as their ethnic status). When I sat in staff meetings taking notes, these were fieldnotes, and I was sitting in those meetings as both a co-investigator and an anthropologist, as a participant as well as an observer.

It was finally agreed that I would receive a list of comments that dealt with what the health professionals saw as partial information, such as a more detailed and nuanced presentation of the place of the experimental carrier matching program within the broader genetics project for which the health professionals were responsible. The ethnographic endeavor is a painstaking, rashomonesque attempt to reconstruct a complex reality out of its multifarious perspectives, and this list of comments indeed helped to clarify important points and massages regarding which I admit to have had partial information. Many of these comments, for which I am grateful, were incorporated into the manuscript. Some of the requests could not be incorporated. The request to refer to all professional respondents as "health professionals," for example, could not be complied with since the reference to respondents as genetic counselors was important in ethnographic terms. As for the negative portrayal of project's staff with which I was imputed, it was agreed that academic freedom should prevail. My reaction to this imputation was actually one of surprise, since it was not my intention to draw a negative portrayal of the project's staff. When working on the manuscript I strove to clarify the complexities of my subjective view regarding the health professionals involved in the experimental program for carrier matching studied here. I do not think these people can be drawn in black or white. They have found themselves in a complex situation without any instruction manuals. Many of the unintended consequences of the carrier matching program were anticipated by the health professionals, but this did not mean that they were fully prepared to deal with those consequences or that they had all the answers. The health professionals' involvement in the carrier matching program was intense and emotional; for many of them it was voluntary; they had well-intended and empathic expectations, and were disappointed when these expectations did not realize. I shared their expectations and disappointments, but I also observed them.

When considering the implications of this experience for applied anthropologists and sociologists in the field of community health care and medical organizations, the major lesson is the importance of daily boundary-work. Apparently it is not sufficient to state one's dual role in a research proposal that represents the espoused theory of the project for purposes of public presentation. The schizophrenic meaning of "participant observation" is not familiar to those outside the field of anthropology and professionals who find themselves turned into researchees are likely to be antagonized. It is essential to negotiate and manage the boundaries between participant and observer on a daily basis, in every meeting and with each respondent. There are additional differences that underpin the organizational culture of the medical profession as opposed to the organizational culture of anthropology and qualitative sociology, and may create misunderstandings and miscommunication. The issue of publication and co-authorship is of course a thorny one in both professions. However the status given to field data seems in my (retrospective) view to be essentially different in medicine and anthropology. What I am about to say is of course a generalization whose external validity requires further evidence. Nevertheless, this hindsight appears to explain some of the conflicts between me and my co-investigators. For the medically-oriented researcher, field data are usually thought to be "owned" by those who were first to publicize them. Once published, they cannot be used again for analysis. This seems to stem from the positivistic and factual status given in biomedical culture to field data. For social scientists, especially those working in the interpretive tradition, this is different. Field data may be repeatedly analyzed and inquired, since they constitute subjective pieces in an interpretive puzzle. When writing this manuscript I did not think about the possibility that by publishing field data on patterns of utilization I would be robbing my co-investigators of the option to use these data in epidemiological papers. Indeed, I still think this data can be differently analyzed from an epidemiological point-of-view, and I do not see my interpretation as being more privileged. These, and other differences that I still may not have understood, should be considered in the context of inter-professional teamwork. I hope this book does not deter readers from such inter-professional endeavors, but rather sharpen their sensibilities to it, as it did for me.

Chapter 3

Biomedical Culture and Ethical Dilemmas: The Professionals' Point-of-View

The six genetic counselors involved in the program consisted of both certified and non-certified counselors. The two certified counselors were Jewish. The four non-certified personnel were Arabic-speaking people with or studying toward academic degrees in genetic counseling, public health, biology or medicine (MPH, MA, MD). Some of them were trained specifically for the program and served as community-outreach assistants. The five professionals directly involved in the program were a medical geneticist, a pediatrician, and three epidemiologists, two of them graduate students who were completing their degrees while working on the administration of the program. In order to secure the anonymity of these respondents, I refrained from adding personal details that could identify them.

The program involved at least three major ethical dilemmas. First, carrier matching raises ethical questions regarding the seeming violation of the patient's lawful right to obtain information about him- or herself. Second, nondirectiveness and patient's autonomy are seemingly compromised by a scheme in which two carriers can be termed "genetically incompatible." Third, the program is ethically questioned by the fact that NSRD is not a severe disease and for many Bedouin (or western people for that mater) would not entail abortion. These dilemmas, as I have noted earlier, do not have clear-cut solutions but rather represent a gray area in which ethical principles acquire new, situated meanings.

The Dilemma of Disclosure

The usual disclosure style in many carrier detection programs is full individual disclosure. While this option existed for the Bedouin, an individual test would cost about $100 (the standard fee for a non-subsidized genetic test), while carrier matching was offered for no charge as part of a budgeted study. The same dilemma existed in *Dor Yeshorim*, the program offered to orthodox Ashkenazi Jews. Israeli geneticists working with *Dor Yeshorim* justified their involvement by claiming that carrier matching was the request of the community. Furthermore, *Dor Yeshorim* was considered by geneticists as "the only way the orthodox community can avoid the agony caused by the birth of babies affected by very devastating diseases" (Sagi, 1998: 427). It was the only way because prenatal diagnosis was irrelevant (due to the religious ban on abortion), and the norm of consanguineous matchmaking was an essential part of life in the community. As one of the counselors said,

> "When you have a group that tells you, in advance, that they're not going to abort, then you have no choice but to do carrier matching. For those people who come for premarital counseling, everything I'll say will be directive. Whatever I say, the question of whether to marry or not to marry would be in the background. Still, I feel that I am keeping my neutrality. I have no dilemma about not disclosing individual information, because those are the rules of the game" (interview #8 with genetic counselor).

As all counselors pointed out, the benefits of carrier matching were directly related to the goals of genetic counseling. The other reason given for supporting carrier matching, namely "the community's will," had its own share of ethical problems. In reality, *Dor Yeshorim*—like other programs in comparable societies—represented the top-down guidance of community leaders (the rabbis), rather than a democratic consensus. The situation was even less clear with the Bedouin, where there was no real leadership—religious or otherwise—and it was very difficult to know "what the community wants."

According to some of the health professionals involved in the program for carrier matching that was offered to the Bedouin, in legal and ethical terms there was not really a dilemma about the patient's right to know. The argument was that patients could always request an individual test, for which, unfortunately, they had to pay, as it (in a similar manner to most other genetic tests) was not part of the health services basket provided by the Ministry of Health. One of the health professionals argued in this context that "the integrative disclosure project is an experimental one. It is funded as a study and not as a public health action. The ethical justification is that patients have the right to know but they also have the right not to know, if they so wish." Testing as part of the program for carrier matching was indeed conditional on signing an informed consent form that explained the rationale of couple screening and in which the individual waived his or her right for personal information. It should be asked, however, whether such consent was really 'informed' and autonomous for both men and women, or whether it was compromised by the medical, economic and socio-political constraints that underpinned this project.

Another important reason given by geneticists and counselors in support of carrier matching stemmed from the potential stigmatization of the carrier in individual disclosure:

> "The ethical justification behind carrier matching is to reduce stigmatization. If just one person in a couple is a carrier, the couple is still said to be genetically compatible. This prevents the labeling of the carrier, labeling that would have taken place in individual disclosure" (interview #5 with genetic counselor).

This argument was supported by statistical computations showing that carrier matching can potentially label one out of 16 of those tested, while individual disclosure can label as many as one out of four (calculated to represent the number of "incompatible" matches and carriers, respectively, per tested people). Stigmatization (particularly of women) could very well take place even with carrier matching. If a match were broken following genetic counseling, rumors would spread around the close-knit Bedouin community, placing a stigma on both sides and particularly on the woman. However, such a scenario could take place only in cases where a match was broken due to "genetic incompatibility." In many other cases, where only one of the mates was found to be a carrier, there would still be genetic "compatibility." In these cases, carrier matching indeed eliminates the burden of stigma from the carrier.

The Dilemma of Nondirectiveness and Autonomy

In an international attitude survey administered to genetic counselors (Wertz, 1998), widespread support was expressed for people's right to choose their mates even if these choices increased their risk of having children with a genetic disorder. The majority of counselors in most nations disagreed with the statement that "people who carry a recessive gene should not mate with another carrier of the same recessive gene" (Wertz, 1998: 502). When presented with the same questionnaire that was used by Wertz, all the counselors involved in the program also disagreed with the above-mentioned statement regarding the restriction of marriage options. However, when we discussed their answers to the questionnaire in an open interview, they acknowledged the gap between this general statement and the actual message characterizing the program. As one counselor said, "This is completely different from what we do in the program. We actually tell people 'you and your mate are genetically incompatible'" (interview #4 with genetic counselor). One of the counselors admitted that she "didn't like the term 'genetic compatibility' and wouldn't have chosen it herself" (interview #8 with genetic counselor).

Another counselor tried to bridge the gap by arguing that

> "While it is true that the bottom line of the counseling consists of whether the partners are compatible or not, we take caution not to say anything about how this affects the prospects of marriage. All we say is that if the partners are genetically incompatible, they should know that they have 25% of having an affected child in each pregnancy, and 75% chance of having a healthy child" (interview #5 with genetic counselor).

However, the counselors knew that because prenatal diagnosis was not a practical option for most couples, the implication of such counseling was "don't marry each other if you don't want to have affected babies" (interview #7 with genetic counselor). This knowledge was also apparent in the attempts of counselors to convince the Bedouin community that the counseling should be done as early as possible in the matchmaking process. "If they do the counseling after the match had been made, there is evidently a greater price for breaking the match" (interview #7 with genetic counselor).

It would be wrong to consider the counselors' attitudes exclusively in the context of abstract ethical reasoning. Their views have also been shaped by past involvement and experience with the Bedouin. Consanguinity, which constitutes—professionally speaking—a "genetic hazard" (interview #2 with genetic counselor), was in this manner accepted, though reluctantly. Moreover, professionals have agreed that "this custom actually provides security for the women, who according to Bedouin culture would lose their children to the husband and his family upon divorce. When cousins marry there is a tendency to solve marital problems within the family and thereby avoid divorce" (Carmi et al., 1998: 393). The early counseling experience with the Bedouin family congenitally afflicted by a lethal metabolic disease is also fundamental to understanding how the principles of the NSRD and thalassemia screening programs were developed. In particular, this early experience provides a clear context for the underlying rationale of "healthy consanguinity." On the one hand, the Bedouin were instructed about the genetic risk of consanguinity; on the other hand, the message of "genetic incompatibility" attempted to be nondirective.

Counselors were quite aware that the formal "nondirective" message of carrier matching was actually interpreted by counselees as a directive for mate selection. This was justified within the constraints of the situation, as seen by the counselors. In the words of one counselor,

> "We keep up with the Bedouin norm of consanguinity, which we all know is responsible for the high prevalence of diseases. We could have told them not to marry their cousins, but we don't, because we know that would be too directive as well as impractical. In the same manner we also keep up with their custom of polygamy, which is quite unacceptable in Jewish or even western eyes. We also understand that their religion does not allow for abortion. All we are left with, then, is the option of premarital testing—and that's what we are doing! Unfortunately it is interpreted as directive, but we have no other option. The alternative is not to do anything. We're damned if we do it, and we're damned if we don't" (interview #2 with genetic counselor).

Another counselor commented that there was not much point in being nondirective when counseling in a population whose own local culture is so directive:

> "Yes, we say in this program 'you don't match in terms of deafness.' It's justified because marriages in the Bedouin sector are mostly prearranged, and because this tribe does not want to have deaf children. Marriage is not about love but about matchmaking. It's not about romance. What they need to do, in the worst case, is to arrange another match. This justifies, for me, the ethical diversion involved in the program" (interview #4 with genetic counselor).

The Dilemma of the Disease's Mildness

The program tested for NSRD, a relatively non-severe disease that for most people would not entail abortion. The counselors basically agreed to this assertion:

> "Deafness is a mild disease compared to what we're usually dealing with in counseling. In addition, there's a treatment in the form of hearing aids or cochlear implantation, which should be covered by the sick funds" (interview #3 with genetic counselor).

Another counselor said:

> "I know of only one case in which there was talk about pregnancy termination due to NSRD. It was a Bedouin woman who already had

> four affected children. She did amniocentesis and the fetus was affected. She wanted an abortion, but her husband did not allow it. I empathized with the woman in this case. It's true I don't think NSRD is severe enough to justify abortion. But I could identify with the woman's situation, her socio-economic predicament. You have to understand her, alone with these kids at home, taking care of them" (interview #2 with genetic counselor).

Another counselor demonstrated the mildness of NSRD through the following story:

> "There was this case with one (Jewish) woman who said she didn't want prenatal diagnosis for NSRD. She told me that 'if it's a deaf child I will not terminate the pregnancy in any event, so why take the test? It will just be more difficult, knowing that the baby is deaf while being pregnant with it.' She preferred to find out about the baby's deafness only after it is born" (interview #4 with genetic counselor).

Counselors therefore acknowledged that NSRD was a mild disease. While they could not solve this dilemma, they framed it as temporary:

> "There are prevalent diseases in the Bedouin population that are much more severe, but we haven't come up with the gene mutation yet. Arthrogryposis, for example. I know they are working on it in the genetic lab" (interview #3 with genetic counselor).

Another counselor acknowledged that

> "NSRD is not the disease I would choose as a basis for such a project to begin with. It's too eugenic. It's a fact, but this fact is rarely brought up when discussing the project. I can understand that NSRD was chosen because of the availability of the mutation and the fact there are so many carriers out there. These are practical reasons" (interview #8 with genetic counselor).

In addition to the major ethical issue of the relative mildness of NSRD, there were several related issues. One related ethical dilemma was whether counselees have been provided with information regarding available treatment and rehabilitation chances, and not just the bleak prospects of the disease. Dunne and Warren (1998), for example, argue persuasively that support foundations must have a stronger voice in the counseling procedure. Rather than being included merely as an afterthought, support foundation personnel must be represented on the health care teams, which deliver results and perform counseling. At the time of the study, the program did not include reference to possible treatments such as hearing aids and implants, and counselors did not mention the possibility of contacting a support foundation for additional information.[9] This was, in the eyes of the professional staff, the role of the audiology institute located at the hospital. Moreover, the general opinion was that implants required a major investment of time and money and continuous inspection that were over-demanding for the Bedouin. In addition, the fact that there was a lack of Arabic-speaking speech therapists and audiologists in the Negev area was evidently also a serious drawback. The Ministry of Education is required to provide speech therapy through the schools for hearing-impaired children. All the schools for the hearing-impaired have part-time speech therapists, but the hours are minimal, averaging 13 minutes a week for each student, and most therapists do not speak Arabic. Only at one Bedouin school is the speech therapist Arabic-speaking, and this is a woman who comes from the North of Isreal two days a week. There are no Bedouin speech therapists, which parallels a great lack of Bedouin professionals in all fields. Speech therapy in particular is problematic because it is considered a woman's profession, women's education is particularly poor, and the necessary training is not yet locally available. This situation means that the program could continue independently of new options that would open up for treatment and rehabilitation. To the outsider, such an attitude might be seen as paternalistic. For the counselors, this attitude was the pragmatic outcome of many years of working with the Bedouin. As one of the program's staff told me,

> "Implantation should not be regarded as a miracle solution. For example, there is currently no Arabic-speaking speech therapist in the entire Negev area. On the other hand, we should do whatever we can to lobby the Bedouin case in conjunction with the sick funds, for maximal coverage of genetic tests and hearing aids."

Another related issue deals with the potentially variable spectrum of the NSRD phenotype. Cohn (1999), as well as other clinical studies of NSRD, reported considerable variation in the degree of residual hearing loss in ho-

9. Interestingly, it is not axiomatic that support foundations should take a moral stand against preventive genetic counseling. Participating as an advisor in discussions for a project that aimed to provide better care for children with hearing impairments, I noticed that the representatives of the Israeli support foundation for hearing-impaired children (MICHA) exclaimed that preventive counseling was a positive thing that should be conducted in tandem with attempts to provide a better care for those affected with a hearing impairment. This issue is further examined in Raz (2004).

mozygotes. While most autosomal recessive disorders have fairly consistent phenotypes, especially within sibships, this is not observed for NSRD; and while these hypotheses are the subject of on-going genetic research, the ethical question is what should be their impact on actual counseling? In genetic disorders that have a spectrum of expression such as Down syndrome or Fragile-X, prenatal counseling should include some reference to the possibility of having a mildly or severely affected child. So far, no variation in the degree of residual hearing loss was found within the Bedouin clan under study. This ethical dilemma was therefore put aside for the time being, as the program was developed and implemented under the assumption that the specific mutation was always expressed, in the recessive homozygote, as profound/severe deafness. New clinical findings could change the existing type of prenatal counseling.

It is interesting to compare the discourse of my professional respondents to that of other geneticists. Kerr et al. (2001), who interviewed a group of geneticists in the UK, argued that these professionals had a negative attitude towards eugenics, and characterized it as politically distorted bad science. The new genetics, in contrast, was presented by British professionals as neutral scientific knowledge and technology, applied to help individuals alleviate genetic disease. These arguments were used together with claims about the public's fear and misunderstanding, and media distortion of the new genetics.

Appeals to individual, informed choice as opposed to coercion were an important way in which the new genetics was distinguished from eugenics. As one of the British geneticists said in the interview:

> "I think my major feeling about that sort of approach to the eugenics question is that we have to keep referring things back to individual choice. I think eugenics for me implies a population, a government, a scientifically led race towards something. I base my practice, and certainly this institution, I'm sure, bases its practice around patient choice. And I think if we aim it at the individual without bias then hopefully we avoid that."

Unlike the Israeli health professionals involved in the genetics program, the British geneticists saw nondirectiveness and individual autonomy as golden standards. The British geneticists ignored the fact that while individual clients of genetic testing may make the ultimate decision concerning their participation, these decisions are embedded in a complex array of familial, cultural, economic, and social experiences and pressures. However, given the backdrop of hostility to people with an increasing array of genetic diseases, clients' choices are far from free. When considered in this way, the line between individual, voluntary choice and socially enforced coercion becomes blurred. It was, indeed, blurred from the point-of-view of the Israeli counselors studied here, but not in the "standard view" of the British geneticists interviewed for a general attitude research enquiry.

In blatant contrast to this "standard view" stands the actual paternalism of UK health professionals interviewed and observed by Darr (1990) in the context of her ethnographic study of thalassemia among British Pakistanis. She quotes the following statements of health professionals (doctors and genetic counselors) about British Pakistanis as typical: "they leave everything to God and don't want to understand or use their initiative"; "they shouldn't marry their cousins. If they didn't, they wouldn't have these diseases"; "their children's health is not a priority with Pakistani parents"; and, the worse statement in Darr's view, "this condition [i.e., thalassemia] was caused by you and your husband being cousins" (1990: 16, 261). These quotes illustrate Darr's serious accusation regarding the inadequate genetic counseling offered to British Pakistanis, which is according to her findings pervaded by ethnocentric cultural assumptions. This description seems a far cry from the attitudes presented by the Israeli genetic counselors and health professionals involved with the Bedouin community. In a parallel manner to the British health professionals studied by Darr, Israeli professionals also felt they were dealing with people who were "different" from them. However, this cultural difference provided an impetus, in the Israeli case, for molding the services to the needs of the population.

Bioethical Criteria for Genetic Screening

Does bioethics have a definite judgement of the dilemmas faced by counselors in the genetics program offered to the Bedouin? One of the acknowledged difficulties in applying ethical principles such as autonomy, beneficence, nonmaleficence and justice, is that there are no definitive criteria to decide which principle is overriding (Chadwick et al., 1999). Another source of criticism, which is very pertinent to our case, is that ethics reflect dominant socio-cultural beliefs, attitudes and values (ten Have and Kimsma, 1990; Hoedemaeker, 1998). In a well-known medical ethics textbook, Beauchamp and Childress (1994: 4) wrote:

> "Often no straightforward movement from theory or principles to particular judgements is possible [....] although general reasons, principles, and even ideals can play some role in evaluating conduct and establishing policies."

The preconditions for community carrier screening, published by the WHO (Modell and Kuliev, 1991) contain the following points:

1. The disease should be a major health problem
2. The course of the disease should be defined (predictable) and severe
3. There must be a simple, accurate, and cheap carrier test
4. There is a solution to the problem
5. There should be educational and counseling backup in the community.

The report of the Nuffield Council on Bioethics (1993) also includes the requirement that the condition should be an important health problem, that there must be an accepted form of treatment, and that the natural history of the condition should be understood. As already mentioned, these recommendations tend to use concepts that allow for different interpretations. For example, what is a serious disease? What is an important health problem? Evidently, value-judgements play a role in such a decision.

Post, Botkin and Whitehouse (1992) suggested (in the context of selective abortion after genetic testing) that three dimensions of the severity of the genetic condition should be considered. These are the degree of harm to health if the disease occurs; the patient's age at onset of the disease (early onset is considered to be more severe); and the probability that people will develop the disease (i.e., the penetrance of the gene). According to their view, the prenatal detection of treatable diseases, late onset diseases, or susceptibilities to diseases does not provide sufficiently weighty reasons to justify abortion.

In other accounts, "severity" has been downplayed in the list of requirements for a worthwhile screening program. For example, in the following scheme that was adapted from Cuckle and Wald (1994), the wording "medically important disorder" replaces "severity":

Aspect	*Requirement*
1. Disorder	Well-defined
2. Prevalence	Known
3. Natural history	Medically important disorder for which there is an effective remedy available
4. Financial	Cost-effective
5. Facilities	Available or easily installed
6. Ethical	Procedures following a positive result are generally agreed and acceptable both to the screening authorities and to the patient
7. Test	Simple and Safe
8. Test performance	Distribution of test values in affected and unaffected individuals known, extent of overlap sufficiently small, and suitable cut-off level defined

Screening for thalassemia arguably fits all the above-mentioned criteria. It is relatively prevalent among a particular sub-population of the Bedouin community, it is severe, and there is a simple test to detect carriers. While thalassemia has early onset and high probability of development, it is nevertheless treatable. Thalassemia patients often live with their disease, although without treatment the disease is serious and leads to early death. In Cyprus, this point has been explained away by pointing to the economic burden of the disease for the community (Hoedemaeker and ten Have, 1998). Screening for NSRD, in Western eyes at least, does not seem to fit the criterion of severity. This brings us back to the dilemma of the disease's mildness, which was indeed raised by the counselors. This dilemma throws into relief the subjectivity of "severity."

The dilemma is not easily solved. There is no bioethical "bottom line" to be offered, since the ethical solution depends on the ethical approach assumed (see Broad, 1930). For example, from a deontological approach—which affirms our capability to establish absolute and exceptionless moral precepts—NSRD screening may be rejected on grounds of the disease's mildness and the overtly directive nature of the program. In contrast, a utilitarian approach to ethics—which considers actions as morally correct when useful for the majority—will justify NSRD screening as promoting the good of community members. Indeed, the prevailing approach to bioethics is utilitarian or consequentialistic: Benefits (such as reducing the incidence of the disease) and harms (such as discrimination, stigmatization, and social pressure) are compared and balanced. If there is a net benefit, genetic testing or screening is thought to be morally acceptable (Hoedemaekers, 1999).

The genetics program studied here presents a complex interface between public and private, professional and layperson, modern and traditional domains. The counselors framed their worries and discords under what they termed as ethical dilemmas. These dilemmas were also directly related to the issue of medicalization. For example, counselors expressed ambivalence in regard to testing for a non-severe condition such as NSRD or using a label such as "genetically incompatible." The ethical dilemmas of counselors show that the biomedical narrative itself is heterogeneous and reflexive. As the program was put in motion, the dilemmas—in a manner typical of organizational dynamics—were gradually submerged by the argument of cultural adaptation.

It is also important to note the impact of the scientific community on local ethical considerations. This is yet another aspect of the institutional analysis of bioethics with which I am concerned in this study. The genetic counselors and health professionals involved in the program subscribed in principle to the "standard ethical code" of genetic counseling. They nevertheless compromised the values of nondirectiveness and individual autonomy when faced with the special circumstances of working with the traditional Bedouin community. When presented to external foundations in order to garner research money, such compromise was often resisted in the grant review process. For example, a comment that repeated itself in several reviews was that while the program emphasized one disclosure style ("integrative disclosure"), in order to be eligible for a grant it should compare the use and implications of this style to other forms of disclosure. Indeed, the health professionals who took the idea of carrier matching ("integrative disclosure") from *Dor Yeshorim* did not (and perhaps could not) subject it to full democratic review by the community. The public meeting that was summoned, for example, included men only, since women are customarily forbidden to attend public meetings together with men.

In a similar manner, one of the reviewers had serious ethical reservations about nondisclosure. This reservation went against the grain of carrier matching, where disclosure is not individual but integrative. Indeed, there can be no "integrative" disclosure without individual *non*disclosure. This principle was borrowed from *Dor Yeshorim* as a way to reduce stigmatization. Nevertheless, the ethical price of nondisclosure was obviously too high for those laboring under a more 'standard view' of bioethics. At this point I do not make any judgement regarding this debate. Rather, I am interested in describing its discursive elements. At the end of the day, the requirements made during the grant review process were therefore one of the factors behind the introduction and implementation of a multiple-step process of community engagement, in which community members reviewed (and could later make use of) various counseling formats.

The Point-of-View of Bedouin Health Professionals

It is widely accepted that the recruitment and training of members of different ethnocultural groups as genetic counselors is an essential component of providing appropriate genetic counseling services to those groups (Weil and Mittman, 1993; Weil, 1998). This is particularly important in the US, given the demographics of genetic counselors—96% Caucasians, 2% Hispanic, 1% African American, and 1% Asian American (Weil and Mittman, 1993: 162). A similar attitude characterized the local genetics institute that served the Bedouin population, where the majority (five out of seven) of practicing (though, indeed, non-certified) counselors were Arabic-speaking, and four were Bedouin themselves. The importance of engaging community members as counselors is not debated in principle. However, my point is that it may not be so simple in practice, as the people involved may experience dilemmas and conflicts. An illustration of the characteristic dilemmas and typical outlook of the Bedouin counselors is provided in the following excerpt. It is taken from an interview conducted with Jamīla (pseudonym), one of the community-outreach counselors, a Bedouin woman in her early 20's with a degree in biology, who worked at the genetics institute for a long period, training to be a certified genetic counselor. She left this course of training owing to what she saw as a religious dilemma. While this particular respondent's decision to quit her training had put her in a unique position, the dilemmas she expressed were nevertheless typical of the rest of the Bedouin who worked at the genetics institute.

Q: "Why were you interested in genetic counseling to begin with?"

A: "Even before I began studying biology, I was interested in genetics. Especially because of the situation in the Bedouin sector, where there are a lot of genetic diseases because of inter-marriage. In my family, too, there is a genetic disease. A few of my relatives have died because of it. I saw genetic counseling as offering information and help."

Q: "Why do you think the custom of inter-marriage is so strong among the Bedouin?"

A: "Because in our sector the family is tied closely together. Our neighborhood, for example, consists of one family. It's not easy to bring a stranger into the neighborhood. People prefer to marry in the family. This way, if there is a problem, it can be solved inside the family, among people who know who you are."

Q: "Is the custom of inter-marriage connected to match-making?"

A: "Yes, traditionally, but today the custom of match-making creates problems. It's like, a son tells his parents he's not going to marry his cousin, even though she had been intended for him. A daughter does not tell her parents something like that, but a son does. And if the son gets his way and marries someone else—this is called romantic love—then his cousin remains single. If a stranger comes to ask for her, her parents would have to say yes, because her cousin already married someone else."

Q: "Did you hear of anyone who was engaged to a cousin and then cancelled the marriage because of genetic counseling?"

A: "No, I didn't. But I know that because I am familiar with the genetic problem, I would not marry my cousin."

Q: "Why cancel the option in advance? You can test first."

A: "No, for me the option of marrying my cousin does not exist in principle. I know there is no test that can tell us we're 100% compatible. There are just specific tests for specific diseases, not all of the diseases. There is a large chance that cousins can create a new disease for their children."

Q: "What about prenatal testing, genetic tests during pregnancy?"

A [excited]: "This is what I told the other counselors, because of this matter of abortions, because according to our religion and according to ethical principles, abortion is forbidden. Some scholars say that it is permitted before 120 days [of gestation]. But for me, as a genetic counselor, if a pregnant woman comes to me and her pregnancy is older than 120 days, I would be obliged to tell her about the test."

Q: "But what if such a woman came to you for counseling, can't you tell her all the information, all the options? Tell her that she can take the test as well as that she can consult a religious guide about it?"

A: "But the problem, according to my religion, is that I should also tell her that abortion is forbidden. If I know that abortion is forbidden, I must tell her. Even if she is secular, or Jewish, I should still tell her that abortion is forbidden."

Q: "What if you ignore the possibility of abortion and just speak to the counselee about the test?"

A: "But if someone does amniocentesis, what do they do it for? It's like even if I don't say the word 'abortion,' it doesn't matter, this is what the test is for. As a genetic counselor, I feel like I am contributing to abortion."

Q: "Did you speak about this with the certified counselor that trained you?"

A: "Yes, I told her that I can do genetic counseling but without the issue of abortion. I can explain about inter-marriage as well as about CVS, because that's an early test. But I cannot explain about amniocentesis and abortions. This is why I left. Because if I work as a counselor, I have to explain about amniocentesis and abortion."

Q: "But if you don't do it, someone else would. I am not trying to influence you in any way, just trying to understand."

A: "Yes, well, it took a lot of time for me to decide that I want to quit. I was in training and was going to do a Master's degree in genetic counseling. I didn't think of any other option, and when I decided to quit, I was left with no other plan. But you have to understand that it was part of a process. During the last year I also became closer to religion. I wasn't dressed like this before." (In the interview, she was dressed with the traditional outfit of an unmarried Bedouin woman, a full-length black robe that leaves only the face unveiled).

Q: "Again, without trying to influence you in any way, I'm interested to hear what you think about the following question. You are a biology graduate. You and I know that the fetus is a living entity as soon as a sperm had fertilized the egg and the zygote starts to develop in the womb. So why do you think that abortion is forbidden only after 120 days?"

A: "Muslim religion claims that before 120 days, the fetus is merely body components without a soul."

Q: "But Muslim religion was written before the advent of modern medicine. Biologically speaking, there is no difference between 119 and 120 days of gestation."

A: "This is how it is. I cannot explain. The *Quran* words are the words of God. It is a spiritual, not a biological thing. What is written in the *Quran* does not depend on changes in human knowledge."

Q: "This makes a lot of sense from a religious point-of-view. What made you come back to religion, if I may ask?"

A: "It's not that I didn't believe before. I believed and all, it was just the traditional dress that was missing. I prayed, I didn't do bad things, the only step was the dress. Then when my religious belief grew stronger I decided it was time to change the dress, too. Even before that, I used to go to meetings with a group of people that spoke about religion, about the end of the world, and about the Day of Atonement. That's when I decided that I have to become fully religious. A friend of mine, who is also religious, asked me about genetic counseling: Do you know if it's all right? How do you do it like that? Then I decided that I should change my dress and quit with counseling."

Q: "What if a friend of yours tells you that she plans to marry her cousin, will you talk to her?"

A: "I always talk about it with friends and relatives. My best friend is half-religious. Her father wanted her to marry her cousin. She said she doesn't want to, she's not sure. She spoke with me about it. She said that she doesn't love him, he's her cousin, and they feel like brother and sister. I explained to her about the genetic risk, the risk of having sick children. In the end, however, she decided to marry her cousin and she didn't do any tests. She studied biology with me, and her cousin was also educated, but nevertheless they got married."

Q: "You're probably familiar with the premarital counseling offered to family X, where hearing loss is prevalent. What do you think of this program?"

A: "I think it's a good program. If someone takes the test and you tell him he is a carrier, he will [....] some people don't understand this thing and they'll think they are sick, it will be like a stigma, if it's a woman people will say 'she's a carrier, don't marry her.' Because people in family X continue to marry inside their family this is a good system for them."

Q: "Do you think they understand what it means to be a carrier? What 'recessive disease' means?"

A: "When I was in training and used to visit the Mother and Child Clinics in the Bedouin settlements, I had to explain to the women about genetic risk. I developed this method to explain about recessive diseases. I would tell them that I have 'gene' in my body [*jinn* in Arabic are spirits that can be either good or bad.] It is hidden and nobody can tell I have it because I'm healthy and can do everything. I can marry someone who has the same gene and he is also healthy, but if both of us give this gene to our child then the child will be sick. I draw it for them, I draw the four possibilities and one of the possibilities is a sick child. One out of four. I have another example for those who don't understand. I tell them, let's say I'm sick and can't wash the dishes at home, my sister will wash the dishes instead. If both of us are sick, who will wash the dishes? No one. This is a funny example, but it helps these women understand the point of a recessive disease. Then I tell them that, if the woman and the man are cousins, then part of their blood is identical, they got it from their grandparents, so if one of the grandparents had the gene, it could have passed down to the cousins. If both cousins have the gene, they have 25% to have a sick child. Sometimes they tell me, I have five healthy children so why do I need this test, so I say that each pregnancy is a different case."

The interview with Jamīla vividly captures the intricacies of the interplay between local Bedouin beliefs and the biomedical premises of genetic counseling. In that sense, the interview provides a glimpse into the complexities of cross-cultural communication on genetic counseling. First, it illustrates the interplay between Muslim religion and genetic counseling. For Jamīla, as well as for many other Bedouin people, being a religious Muslim entailed a ban on abortion. In a similar vein, Islam has a restraining influence on birth control, and conservative Muslim religious leaders frequently oppose the concept. Despite theological interpretations which under certain circumstances may permit the use of contraception, many are more likely to accept the conservative view since large families are the prevailing norm (Azaiza, 1996; Omran, 1993). Abortion is a complex subject in Muslim law, and is legally judged "reprehensible." This means that it is permitted only when a "good" reason can be furnished, and only up to 120 days into the pregnancy, which is the stage before ensoulment. Only when the continuation of pregnancy endangers the mother's life is abortion permitted later than 120 days of pregnancy (see Rispler-Chaim, 1999; Rogers, 1999). This position has vague support in the *Quran*, is explicitly spelled out in *hadith* (narratives of the Prophets' life), and has a direct legal application for inheritance, the determination of blood money in case of injury leading to miscarriage, and in burial rites. Why was the period of 120 days chosen as the point of ensoulement? The answer is given in the following *hadith* (cited in Rogers, 1999:126):

> Abdullah said that the Prophet of God (may peace and blessings be upon him) said that the sperm is in the womb for forty days without its condition changing. When it has passed these forty days it becomes a clot, then in that manner it becomes a bigger thing likewise, and when Allah wants to complete its creation, He sends an angel. He tells the angel that which He commands for it: for example, male or female, unhappy or joyful, short or tall, weak or strong, and he makes the person healthy or infirm. He (the Prophet) said that he (the angel) writes all of this down [...]

The Muslim description of creation within the womb thus falls into two major stages, marked by the line of 120 days. The most common prenatal genetic test, amniocentesis, is performed after 16 gestational weeks (112 days) and an additional three weeks are required for cell growth in the laboratory. This means that amniocentesis results are available too late (i.e., after 120 days). Another prenatal genetic test, CVS, can be performed earlier—in the 11th gestational week.

Other Bedouin individuals who worked in the genetics institute as community-outreach assistants said they could understand and identify with Jamīla's dilemma, but that they were not as religious as she was. Nevertheless, another Bedouin community-outreach counselor called Jasmine (pseudonym) told me (personal interview) that for her "it is also difficult to tell counselees about amniocentesis. I wouldn't do amniocentesis myself because the answer is given too late [for abortion]. I think it would be a good idea to publicize the possibility of the early test, CVS." Other Bedouin health professionals, however, said that the community was not aware of the 120 days *fatwa* (religious instruction), and that abortion was considered reprehensible at any time of pregnancy. The Jewish counselors told me that it was agreed that those community-outreach counselors, who did not feel comfortable about it, would not mention prenatal testing. Counselees who were referred to the institute would hear about prenatal testing there, from the senior counselors. This strategy was evidently not satisfactory for Jamīla. When I asked Jasmine how she felt about Jamīla's decision, she said:

> "I have lots of support at home. My father told me that I have a future in genetic counseling and that it is better than working at school as a teacher. My father is religious, but it doesn't bother him. Jamīla and me, we are good friends. She told me that she doesn't see any future for her in counseling. She prefers to be a schoolteacher. You have to understand the difference between us. Jamīla is not married. I am. She comes from a settlement that is not as liberal as my hometown. When

> we studied for a degree in biology at the university, I lived in the students' dormitory, but she couldn't. Her father didn't let her and she had to go home every day. It was very difficult for her to get to all those Bedouin settlements in which we had to work, because she doesn't have a driver's license and she had to get there by public transportation."

There was a consensus among the Jewish counselors and other professionals, all of them secular individuals, that Jamīla's decision to quit was an unfortunate in terms of the service provided for the Bedouin community, but that it was obvious that Jamīla could not continue as a counselor. When the issue of Jamīla's decision to quit was discussed in a meeting of the steering committee, one of the Jewish counselors who trained Jamīla explained that Jamīla's decision was the result of "social pressure" from the community. In the counselor's words,

> "Jamīla was influenced and converted back to Islam. Other Bedouin women that are working for us also started to think about it. Women are more susceptible to such pressure than men. I suggest we find a man for this job."

In the counselor's view, Jamīla—as a young Bedouin woman looking to find a husband—faced pressure from her family who told her that her marriage prospects will decrease as a genetic counselor because this line of work goes against the religious norms of the community. While this explanation could be valid, it nevertheless also represented a shift of emphasis from Jamīla's individual free will to the "collective imperative" ('mentality' was the word used in the meeting) of the Bedouin community.

There was also a consensus among counselors and professionals that CVS needed to be offered to the Bedouin as soon as possible. There was even an initiative to photocopy a poster containing a *fatwa* (religious instruction) regarding the 120 days ban alongside information about the early use of CVS, and post it in Mother and Child clinics in Bedouin settlements. This poster, Jewish professionals argued, could be used by nurses and community-outreach assistants in order to familiarize Bedouin women with the early prenatal test. This idea was not implemented because of the problems perceived to be associated with CVS use. CVS is currently offered at the local hospital only to families who are at high risk for severe diseases as the risk for miscarriage in CVS is twice as high as in amniocentesis. According to health care professionals, CVS cannot be offered on a wide basis because it must be performed at a very early stage of pregnancy, before most women register for prenatal care. So far, only few families have used this procedure. Although CVS could provide a solution, in theory, to the issue of the 120 days, health professionals were skeptic about it owing to the fact that most Bedouin women do not register for the early prenatal care required for CVS referral, as well as due to the increased risk for miscarriage entailed by CVS.

A second theme in Jamīla's interview is the interplay between consanguinity, matchmaking and the value of genetic counseling. Jamīla's religious beliefs, which made her uncomfortable in the role of a genetic counselor, also led her to stress the important function of premarital carrier matching. Her comments illustrate her conclusion that given the existence of a ban on abortion and a pervasive custom of consanguinity, carrier matching was the only remaining option. In that sense, Jamīla's views and the counselors' view of "healthy consanguinity" converge rather than diverge.

A third theme in the interview is concerned with the interplay between endogenous frames of mind and biomedical models. Jasmine (pseudonym), the other Bedouin community-outreach counselor, told me (personal interview) that she explained the carrier concept as "a person that has the gene for the disease." In her words, "I explain that marrying your cousin causes a genetic risk because you marry 'near at hand blood' and there is an increased risk that carriers will come together." Jasmine used a version of Jamīla's story in explaining that "when two women work together, they finish the house chores in 20 minutes. When one is sick and the other is working alone, it takes her at least 40 minutes. If both are sick, nobody does the work. The same goes for carriers. A carrier has one gene that is sick. It's working, but slowly. Someone who has two sick genes, is altogether sick."

While medically incorrect, the images and stories used by Bedouin assistant counselors to explain the notions of "carrier," "recessive," and "genetic risk" perform an important function of cultural translation. A key concept in the diffusion of global and local cultures is that of hybridization (Hannerz, 1992, 1996), which can also characterize the local translation of global biomedicine. Lim Tan (1989) described the widespread acceptance of the antibiotic Terramycin in rural Brazil. Popular adoption of antibiotic therapy led to this antibiotic being called *Terramicino di Mato,* i.e., "herbal" Terramycin. In this process, the local population domesticated modern and unfamiliar biomedicine in order to make it seem culturally acceptable. Lim Tan's assumption was that such processes are symptomatic of "transitional" medical systems, which develop within what he called "transitional" societies, societies in the process of becoming modern. In another study, Delaney (1991) described how villagers in Turkey adopted the use of 'blood' as a key symbol for heredity following a governmental health campaign. However, contrary to scientific discourse, the local use of "blood" represented the belief that the child's important traits are inherited from the father. The common image of the father who "plants the seed" and the mother as providing "the soil" supports this view (Delaney, 1991; Fedida, 1984). In a parallel manner, the Bedouin worldview also considers blood ties to be primarily agnatic or patrilineal (Kressel, 1992). Female blood ties are regarded as weaker than male or agnatic kinship (Abu-Lughod, 1986). The process of cultural translation evidently does not involve just the health professionals. I will further discuss it in the following chapter, which deals with the utilization of the program and the attitudes of community members.

The views of Bedouin health professionals were far from uniform. Jamīla's attitude, as we saw, represented a relatively extreme identification with the religious norms of the Bedouin community. In contrast, the other Arab and Bedouin individuals kept their involvement in the program out of pragmatic and professional interests. Dr. Taabet (pseudonym), a Bedouin physician who was a member of the steering committee of the program, represented quite an opposite point-of-view, as illustrated in the following excerpt taken from an interview with him.

Q: "What is your involvement in the program for reducing hereditary diseases among the Bedouin?"

A: "I am involved in this research since about 1992, when the first genetic studies were conducted among the Bedouin. After we had the mutation and the epidemiological data, we wanted to convey the message to the young Bedouin generation, to help them think about a new direction. According to Bedouin tradition it is very hard to say I don't want to marry inside the family. We couldn't give them such directions because this would have led to difficult problems. So, we figured, let's do something unique, that has been done in the orthodox Jewish community, let's tell them to think about pre-marital testing, before they get married, before they are even engaged."

Q: "You are talking about family X."

A: "No, in general. I don't want to mention names. We started with a certain family, a certain clan that is quite large, and has the highest prevalence of consanguinity in Israel, second and third wife marriage are also very prevalent, therefore we figured that since we discovered their mutation we can offer the test to the population. In practice, two people take the test and see if they match genetically, if they don't then they can find someone else in the family. In this way at least we contribute to marriage of people that are not both carriers. This was the goal. But then we had to figure out a way of implementing it. It is impossible in such a tribe to go from house to house and offer them a genetic test. However we started doing such a thing. In any event you have in this area over 100,000 Bedouin and not just that tribe. So, we thought about making a film, showing it on TV, and at schools, especially to the young generation."

Q: "What is your opinion about Bedouin consanguinity?"

A: "I think it is a bad thing. It is an old and crooked tradition. All this tribal racism, and I call it racism, it separates rather than unites our people. It causes separatism in the Bedouin population. Separatism is wrong in every society. There are certain Bedouin families who consider themselves better in terms of social standing and consider other as inferior. This is the source of never-ending feuds and quarrels. Every week you can hear about a Bedouin who got wounded or killed because of this. We are living in 2000, but this situation still pervades our society. I ask myself, have we made any progress? If a Bedouin goes to the university but retains his traditional mentality then he doesn't know where to put his diploma. It is just a piece of paper on the wall. It is not enough to make economic progress, to have a car and a house and a degree. You must make mental progress too. I say that tradition and modern culture do not fit."

Q: "You said the younger generation should be the main target. But traditionally it's the parents who decide about the match, isn't it?"

A: "It is always necessary, for change to happen, that someone will demolish the boundaries of the past. If the youngsters don't break the ways of the old, when will they change? You can change only when you're emotionally involved. This is our task: To get the youngsters emotionally involved in this program. But I have to say something: This is not going to happen in the near future. It will take years. 50 years ago when the state of Israel drove away some of the Bedouin, or you can say that some Bedouin have fled across the borders, never mind the circumstances, Bedouin people used to marry without boundaries then. Today they don't. And when the state built new settlements for the Bedouin, they made them like ghettoes, built around specific families in closed quarters. How can they see other families, how can young men meet young women that are not from their family? They have no other option but to marry inside the family."

Q: "This research has a strong element of intervention. How do you account for it, ethically speaking?"

A: "Ethically speaking I don't feel like I'm out of line. On the contrary, I think compelled to help the population. As a member of this population, it is my ethical duty to explain the facts. Explaining can be done in many ways, in the clinic, in a film, and so on. If I don't start doing it, nobody will. Others in the sector do not know the genetics. I did the studies. It is very important for the population to know the information. It's something they never realized. Of course it is very important not to give out names. Nobody likes to be called sick. But we should make the population aware about how many children die every year from hereditary diseases. Compared to the Jewish population, the Bedouin child mortality is about threefold! Why? The first reason is consanguinity. The population needs to know these things. So in terms of ethics, my commitment is to help. In the program we're doing, in which we tell people whom to marry, we don't tell them who's sick. I just tell them if they're compatible or not. I will never tell them who's the carrier."

Q: "This can perhaps work in case they're compatible but if they're not then you're putting the blame on both, actually."

A: "Well, people need to help themselves. I cannot say that someone is a carrier. After they receive the information from me, if the person starts to tell people we're not compatible and starts to publicize it, this is his problem. But anyway people are not ready to take the test yet. It's a difficult process. It doesn't proceed easily. It takes time. About a week ago someone came to see me about taking the test before getting married. For me, this was like Nobel Prize, this is great."

Q: "What about informed consent? Population consent?"

A: "I have to tell you about population consent, I think I'm to blame for that. The population sees me as one of its own. When they saw I was in the program, then they believed us. It is blind faith, and this is consent."

The issues that emerge in the interview with Dr. Taabet relate to his views on consanguinity, the implementation of the program, and the Bedouin people in general. Another major theme, which runs through the entire interview and underpins Taabet's views, is his dual position as a Bedouin and a doctor; "between two worlds," in his own definition. Dr. Taabet's analysis of consanguinity raises the issue of Bedouin "separatism" (in his terms). His "macro" view stresses the negative implications of this system as a barrier to modernity. This contrasts with the "micro" view expressed by Jamīla, the Bedouin assistant counselor who quit the program. Jamīla explained the strength of consanguinity by stressing that "the family is tied closely together [...] People prefer to marry in the family. This way, if there is a problem, it can be solved inside the family, among people who know who you are." Both views, evidently, are equally "authentic" and their co-existence should alert us to the gendered and heterogeneous construction of Bedouin culture.

In his interview and general involvement, Dr. Taabet presented himself as an avid supporter of the program. This support is rhetorically constructed and accounted for, in the interview, through two different knowledge claims: genetic and cultural. Taabet presents his views as stemming from his professional proficiency in genetics and medicine as well as his familiarity with Bedouin culture. This combined authority lends legitimacy to his criticism, which the other (Jewish) program members may have shared but did not express in public. Taabet's "modern" criticism of Bedouin consanguinity as backward, separatist and "racist" custom is an example. Many studies have documented the linkage between biomedicine and modernization or even colonialism (see Comaroff and Comaroff, 1992, 1997; Navarro, 1986; Waitzkin, 1983). The attitude of Dr. Taabet is reminiscent of colonial missionaries and medical troops that set out to 'civilize' the 'primitives.' He speaks for "the Bedouin" as well as for "modern culture." In many discussions of the steering committee, when one of the professionals asked "but what will the Bedouin say?" Dr. Taabet would naturally offer his view about the Bedouin answer. The project staff, it needs to be stressed, did not take for granted views expressed by Bedouin professionals as expressing or representing the Bedouin community. Taabet's paternalism was expressed in speaking for an entire population out of an ideology that was assumed to be objectively progressive. This is why Taabet asserted in the interview that he should "take the blame" for compromising the principle of consent. Although well intended and backed by professional expertise, this was, nevertheless, paternalism.

Chapter 4

Utilization and Attitudes: The Bedouin Point-of-View

At the time of the study about 60% of all clan members had received instruction and about 250 blood samples have been drawn. Those tested were usually unmarried community members around 13–17 years old. Their father signed for their informed consent. The instructions were delivered to extended families and all those attending were counted as having been instructed. Six counseling sessions have so far taken place as part of the program, with six more individual counseling sessions. To assess the prevalence of consanguinity in this clan, a local marriage registrar in the clan was consulted and his records showed that the number of new marriages was 57 during the period of 1999-2002. It should be noted that not all married couples register (for example, according to the registrar polygamous marriages are usually not registered) and this number is therefore probably lower than the actual number of marriages. However, this record can still serve as an indication of the rates of consanguinity. 51 of these marriages (89%) were consanguineous, with 21 (37%) being double first-cousin marriages, 12 (21%) first-cousin marriages, 7 (12%) uncle-niece marriages, 5 (9%) marriages of first cousins once-removed, and 6 (11%) second-cousin marriages. Approximately similar frequencies of double first-cousin marriage, which is the preferred pattern of endogamy among the Bedouins, were found in other studies conducted in the larger Bedouin population (Weitzman et al., 2000). The percent of counseled couples and individuals (out of the total number of annual marriages) was about 20%. So far, no couple was found to be "genetically incompatible." It is still unknown whether in such a case the match would actually be broken, or not. The genetics program for thalassemia, offered to another Bedouin sub-population, is regarded by counselors as being still in the stages of community engagement and instruction. The small number of people seeking counseling was explained by counselors as reflecting the program's early stage of implementation. Counselors expected that the numbers of people seeking counseling will gradually increase as children whose blood was drawn will come of age and consider marriage in the future.

During the program's implementation there have been no cases of amniocentesis in the clan targeted for NSRD testing. The overall uptake of amniocentesis in the Bedouin population is, indeed, very low (about 3% per annum or 31 cases per 1,104 Bedouin women who gave birth, all of them women over 35 years of age; see Weitzmann et al., 2000). In the thalassemic sub-population there have been three cases of young couples who went to a hospital in Tel-Aviv for CVS. This was done without informing their parents. In all cases, the fetus was not affected.

The small number of people seeking counseling, explained by counselors as reflecting the program's early stage of implementation, was possibly also a result of the relatively non-severe nature of congenital hearing loss, or NSRD. Nevertheless, it appears that a specific pattern of utilization has emerged during the program's early implementation. Only long-term research spanning around 20 years can determine the success or failure of such a program. However, I believe it is intriguing to examine those data which are presently at hand. The pattern that characterizes the first (and formative) years is no doubt important in highlighting the weaknesses and strengths that will continue to influence the program as it unfolds.

Following the meetings and discussions, at-home instructions in Arabic were offered to the Bedouin. Instructions typically lasted around three hours, were given in the guest room of the house (*shiqq*) and included basic genetic information and explanations regarding carrier matching. The instructors also explained the informed consent forms and coordinated a date for blood drawing. This chapter first provides a detailed socio-demographic description of the population and then describes the reception of the program's implementation by that population. In doing so my focus will be on the Bedouin clan afflicted by NSRD, where patterns of utilization have already begun to take place.

Basic Information Regarding Consanguinity Levels, Education, Religiosity and Prevalence of Genetic Testing

The following information was collected from a large sample (about one third of the targeted population): Age, gender, marital status, education, religiosity, familial proximity to affected individuals, and utilization of genetic testing/counseling were surveyed. The surveyed sample consisted of 932 clan members (421

Table 1. Educational Levels in the Targeted Population

Years of Education	Male %	Female %
0	6.2	19.9
1	0.7	0
2	2.7	3.7
3	12.3	7.5
4	15.1	11.2
5	12.3	3.7
6	4.8	1.9
7	3.4	3.1
8	15.1	13.0
9	6.2	12.4
10	2.1	1.9
11	3.4	2.5
12	7.5	4.3
13	1.4	1.2
14	0	0.6
15	0.7	3.1
16	4.8	0
17	0.7	0
20	0.7	0
Total	100.0	100.0
Mean	6.7	5.76

males and 511 females) and was drawn from the records of at-home instructions conducted by community-outreach assistants with Bedouin families in the clan as part of the implementation of the genetic counseling projects.[1] In regard to education, an average of 6.73 years of education was found for men and an average of 5.76 years of education was found for women (see table 1).

These figures represent a tremendous change, relatively speaking, in the education of the young generation. Dinero (1997) found in a general survey that 77.8% of the Bedouin fathers (older generation) had no education, and 12.3% had some elementary education. The education of girls, in particular, presents a significant development in resettled Negev Bedouin society. Similar studies covering the entire Bedouin community cite higher secondary school figures (10% graduating), but lower college figures (0.6% with a university degree). These statistics may be compared with 47% high-

1. Data on this sample was collected by Marcela Atār as part of her doctoral research on genetic counseling to the Bedouin, which she is conducting under my supervision. Marcela also performed the statistical analyses on this data, and contributed to my thinking through her methodological skills and theoretical insights.

Table 2. Prevalence and Degree of Consanguinity in the Study Group

Degree of Consanguinity	Frequency	Percent
1st Degree	31	26.7
2nd Degree	15	12.9
3rd Degree	18	15.5
4th Degree	12	10.3
None	40	34.5
Total Marriages	116	100.0

school graduates and 8% university graduates for all Israelis (Dinero, 1997). Male respondents in the sample were far more likely to have attended school and to be literate than female respondents and younger respondents were predictably more educated than older respondents.

Within the 116 marital bonds in the sample, 66% of all marriages were consanguineous with 27% being cousin marriage (first degree consanguinity, in genetic terminology); only 34% of the marriages were not consanguineous at all (see table 2). This provides yet another indication of the high rates of consanguinity in this Bedouin community. It should be noted, however, that most consanguineous marriages were not between cousins, but were more commonly other forms of consanguinity.

67.8% of the sample had some family relation to NSRD. In terms of religiosity, the majority (55.8%) regarded themselves as traditional, 25% as orthodox and 19.2% as secular. Out of the sample, 107 people took the genetic test (61 men, 46 women). The distribution of ages of those who took the test is shown in table 3. The majority of those tested were 13–17 year old, which is the general age period for premarital engagement (see table 3).

The research assistant and I were first tempted to statistically examine the association between social parameters such as consanguinity levels or education, and the use of genetic tests. Indeed, the association between parents' degree of consanguinity and whether their children were genetically tested was found to be significant and positive. This finding could be seen as supporting

Table 3. Distribution of Age in Tested Individuals

Age	Frequency	Percent
13–17	56	52.3
18–22	37	34.6
23–32	12	11.3
33 and up	2	1.8
Total	107	100.0

the Health Belief Model prediction, since consanguinity is supposed to reflect susceptibility, and those who are more susceptible are expected to use genetic testing. However, there was a blind spot in this interpretation. Consanguinity level was *an objective index*. It was not necessarily equivalent to a *subjective perception* of susceptibility. The association between consanguinity and genetic testing should therefore be explored using qualitative, ethnographic methods. In the following sections I turn to describe the specific components of the program from the point-of-view of the clients.

The Instruction Session

The component of instruction was an important intermediary phase before testing and counseling could take place. About 120 instruction sessions have taken place so far with families. Each session took about 3–4 hours and was conducted in the family's home. The two instructors, both in their thirties, were a local Bedouin man whom I will call Yusuf and an Arab woman whom I will call Kadiya, who was working as a school teacher. Usually the two of them cooperated during the instruction session, thus allowing for a mixed audience of men and women to be present. Many of the sessions, it should be noted, took place only after numerous cancellations. Despite daily confirmations and re-confirmations (made via cellular phones[2]), the instructors have traveled many times to the village in the scheduled day, only to find that the parents were gone. I provide here a detailed description of one typical instruction session, conducted in August 1999. This session is characteristically divided into four stages: (1) social introduction and name taking, (2) informative explanations, (3) questions and answers, and (4) sign-up for blood drawing. In addition to describing the general structure of the instruction session, I use this particular description to highlight the interplay between Bedouin attitudes and the process of medicalization.

Leaving the driveway and going down a bumpy road, Kadiya's car entered the shantytown, an unrecognized village with a third-world appearance. Families lived in clusters, there were no streets and we depended on our guides to find the way. We arrived at Salem's house (all names have been changed), where the instruction took place inside the "guest room" (*shiqq*), a separate building of cement blocks with a carpet-covered floor and an asbestos roof.

2. Since the tribe resides in an unrecognized village there are no telephones in the homes. Far from being a status symbol, the abundance of cellular phones in the tribe simply represents the lack of regular telephones.

The family that sat with us included Salem's mother, his two wives, six sons and five daughters (three of them congenitally hearing-impaired). Salem sat near the instructors together with his sons. All the women sat together in the far corner of the room. Salem's younger brothers and his father, who lived nearby, did not come to the instruction.

Kadiya, the female instructor, began by writing down the names of all family members. Yusuf, the male instructor, explained to me that it was usually Kadiya who filled the names because despite his familiarity with the community, he did not remember all the exact names, and asking would make him lose face. In addition, Kadiya usually invited the women and daughters to join in the guestroom (traditionally a male territory), an invitation which, coming from Yusuf, would be impolite. After all names were written down and refreshments (black coffee, tea and fruit) taken, the instruction started.

Yusuf and Kadiya have established a pre-arranged division of labor, which the following description reflects. Yusuf started by introducing the program, noting its official sponsors (the Ministry of Health and the Genetics Institute). Kadiya then proceeded with the explanations, using a pre-prepared kit of flip charts with various Mendelian diagrams and other illustrations with Arabic captions.

The charts were based on the conventional human genetics curriculum taught in highschool. Special attention was given, during the translation of the charts, to avoid any stigmatic reference to carriers and affected individuals. Indeed, the drawings in the flip chart were different from their counterparts in the school curriculum. The school curriculum contained, for example, a conventional depiction of a family tree for the illustration of Mendelian inheritance (figure 1). In this depiction, the affected baby is black, the healthy baby (called "normal") is white, and the carriers are gray. Given the symbolic connotation of white as pure and black as filthy, this graphic depiction could be seen as stigmatic, and was hence rejected by the program's staff. Another diagram in the school curriculum illustrated a "typical Bedouin family tree" depicting the "characteristic phenomenon" of the expression of the recessive disease following numerous cousin marriages (figure 2). According to one of the counselors, the description attached to the drawing was in itself stigmatic, although scientifically correct. Once again, the affected individuals were blackened. The message was further illustrated by a simpler diagram depicting the birth of an affected child as the result of cousin marriage. The health professionals noted that the affected child's image was enlarged and his body proportions convoluted (figure 3). All these depictions were removed from the flip chart since they were considered too stigmatic for presentation during at-home instruction.

Figure 1: Diagram of Mendelian Heredity of Recessive Traits

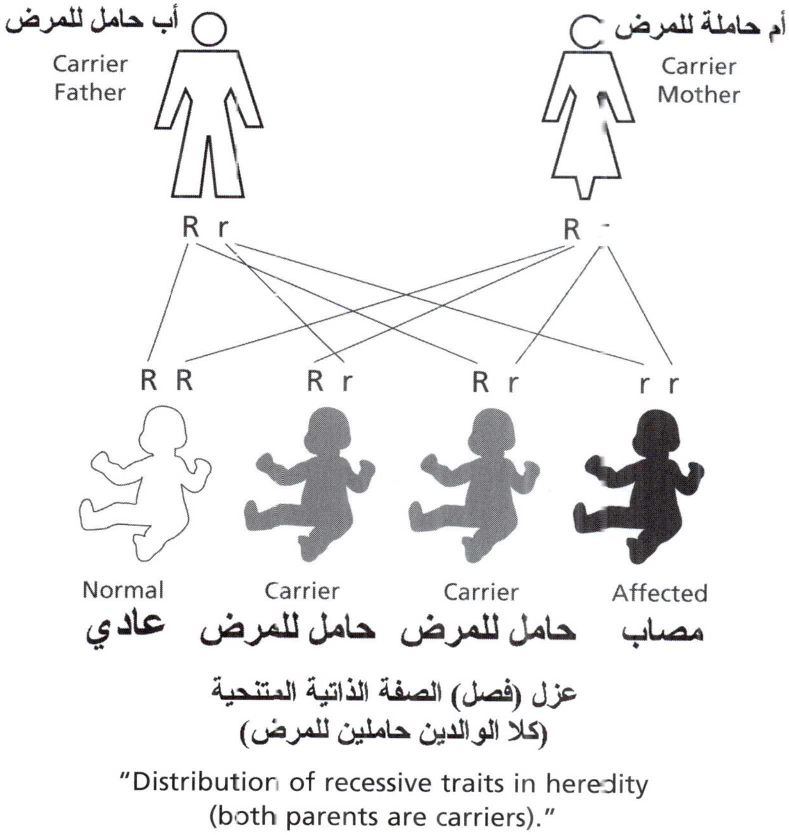

The new set of drawings that was used in the flip chart emerged from a group-concerted effort involving creative imagination. The program's staff debated, for example, how to graphically represent the mutation of the carrier. One suggestion was to draw two copies of the gene with one of the copies (the "mutation") marked by an X. The objection was that such an X would be the graphic equivalent of something bad and defective, and hence should be avoided. One of the health professionals commented in this context: "I have a problem with marking the defective gene on people. This is why I think we should take out the gene and put it outside the body. If I put in on people's body, I feel like I'm marking them." Another suggestion was to locate the graphic depiction of the mutation on or connected to the affected bodily spot. For example, it was suggested to draw a depiction of the mutation inside a cir-

Figure 2: Diagram of a "Typical Bedouin Pedigree," Illustrating the Linkage between Consanguinity and Recessive Diseases

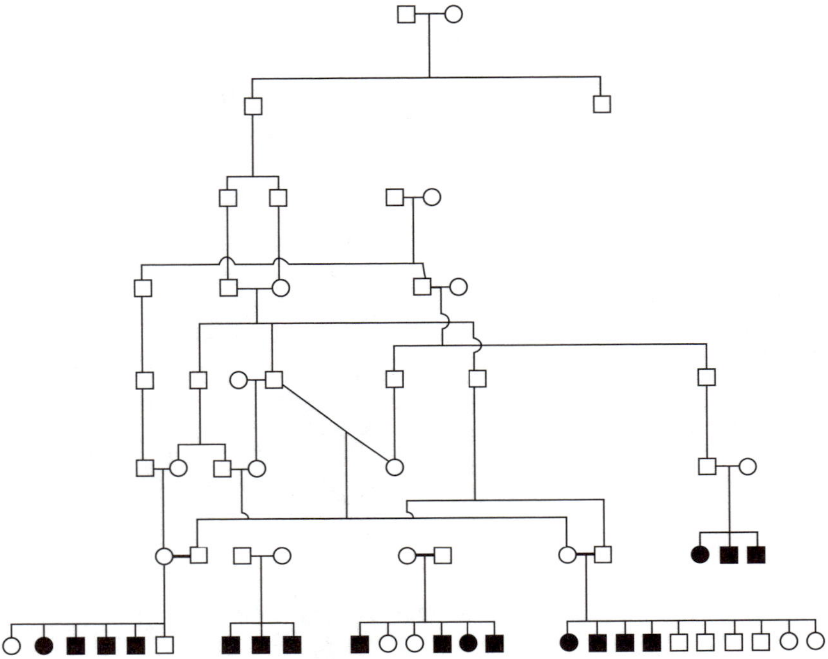

cle connected to the ear, thus creating a visible and symbolic connection between the mutation and congenital deafness. The objection was that such a drawing would again create a linkage between carrier status and the disease. The final image that appears in the flip chart depicts the mutated gene copy outside the body using a "neutral" mark (rather than an X). The circle containing the "genes" was connected to a general point in the center of the chest (figure 4).

Using the flip chart, Kadiya began with general genetics, stating that genes determine the composition of our body. She then moved on to Mendelian genetics, explaining that genes are received from both parents. The concepts of recessive and dominant genes were then explained using the example of

Figure 3: Diagram of First-Cousin Consanguinity with an Affected Child

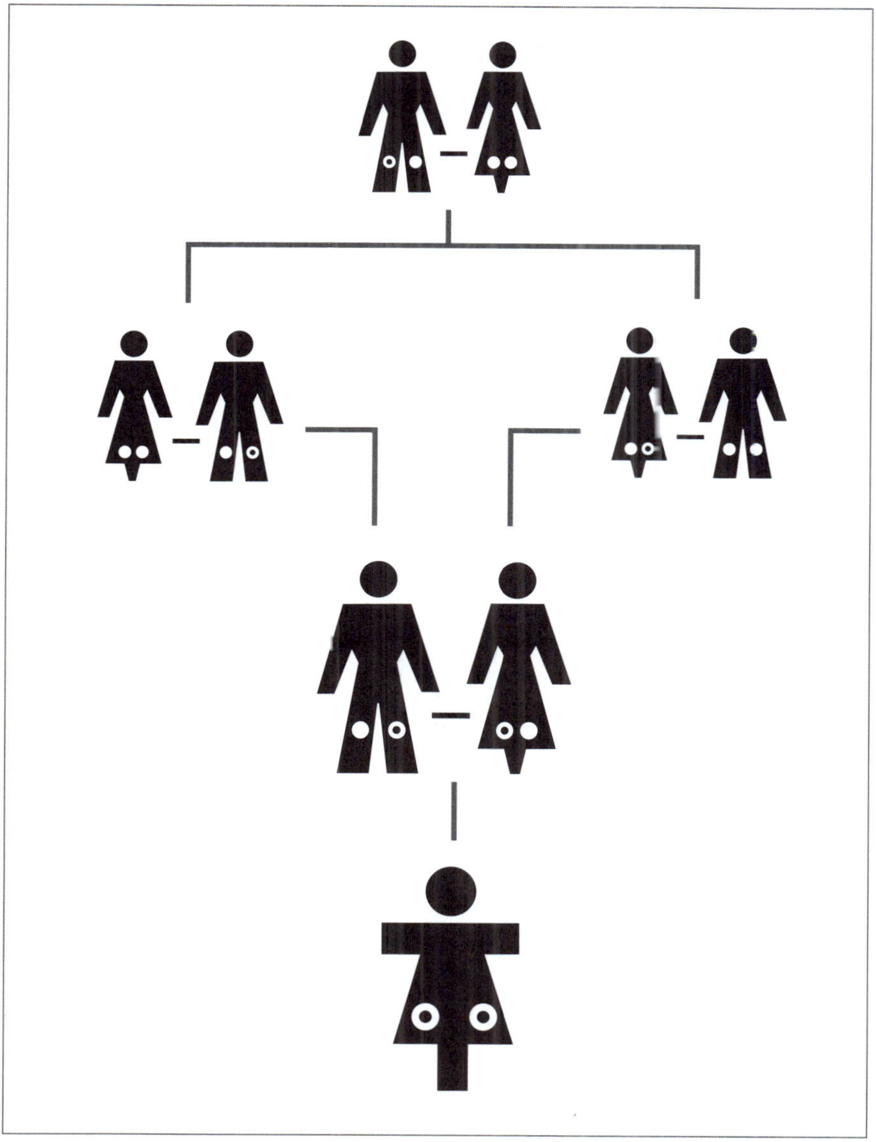

Figure 4: Depiction of Mutation in Flip-Chart for Instruction

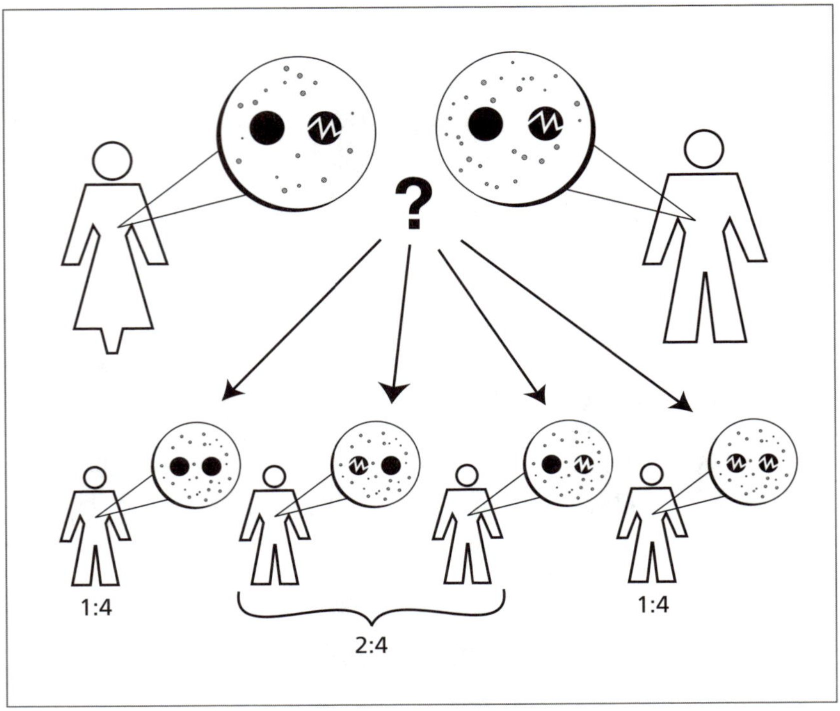

brown/blue eyes. "Brown is stronger than blue, therefore it dominates," Kadiya explained. Deafness, she said, was quite like eye color. The following illustration in the flip chart depicted the four possible combinations of two parental genes—one called in Arabic "*jinn el-haras*" (deafness gene) and the other "*jinn el-saama*" (hearing gene).[3] Yusuf replaced Kadiya and explained about the probabilities of having a deaf child. Salem recognized his family in the flip chart, having understood that since he had deaf children, therefore he and their mother (his first wife) must be carriers.

3. In Bedouin interpretation, this combination could be literally understood as 'the spirits (*jinn*) of deafness' and 'the spirits of hearing.'

He then asked his first wife: "Why couldn't you give all our children the good gene?"
And she replied: "Why couldn't you?"
Kadiya interfered and said: "It came from both of you—fifty fifty."
The whole exchange was spoken in light tone and Kadiya's final remark was received with brief laughter. Yusuf then explained about the program's confidentiality, and the phases of blood drawing, coded storage and carrier matching. It was late in the evening and two young children have fallen asleep.

The third stage of the session commenced with few questions coming from Salem and his two wives. Some of the questions were technical, for example: How old should a child be to qualify for the test? When there were no more questions, Kadiya asked Salem for his ID and wrote down his and his family members' details. Salem and his wives then signed an informed consent form. It was in Hebrew and they did not bother to read it, but rather received a short explanation in Arabic. Addressing the two instructors, Salem asked that his second wife be tested.
"I want to know if she's a carrier," he said, "because I don't want any more deaf children. I already have two healthy children from her, she's young and can have many more."
Yusuf's reply was: "For such an individual test you cannot use the program. You have to take her yourself to the Institute [for testing and counseling]."
Salem said he would.
I asked him what would happen if his wife were found to be a carrier.
His reply was, "then we will do the test in each pregnancy."
Kadiya told me later, in the car, that he was actually saying that abortion was a possibility. But, she added, "we cannot discuss it in the instruction."

Salem's case presents a positive and rational attitude towards genetic testing, which leads to dual utilization (using the program for his children and an individual test for his second wife), a pattern that was found in other cases, too. This was received with mixed feelings by the program's staff. On the one hand, it was an indication of utilization by community members. It was a sign that genetic counseling can serve a useful purpose for the community. On the other hand, it was feared that if the wife were found to be a carrier, her husband would "solve the problem" by taking another wife. Notwithstanding Salem's "promise" to do a prenatal test in each pregnancy if his wife were found to be a carrier, experience has shown that in other, similar situations, the result was taking a new wife. Genetic counseling could therefore inadvertently contribute to the stigmatization of the carrier wife and, consequently, to polygyny. Health professionals deemed both of these consequences negative. Indeed, the system of carrier matching was conceived precisely in order to avoid such consequences. However, it was the counselors' view that such individual requests for "wife-testing" could not be rejected, either on legal grounds or without compromising the principle of individual autonomy. The irony of these cases was that the husband already violated the (Western) principle of autonomy. The wives were often very reluctant to take the test, but did not dare to refuse their husband. This was an example of the "unintended consequences" of the program, once it was put in motion.

In the car, driving back to Beer-Sheva, Kadiya and Yusuf concluded that the visit went well. They compared it to more difficult "cases" of old tribesmen who refused to meet for instruction. In Yusuf's words, "Some old people say it's all in the hands of *Allah* (God) anyway. Their children want to participate but they forbid them. We call on them four times and more. The first time, we speak outside the house. The second time, we enter 'just for coffee.' The third time they let us show the pictures [flip chart]. The fourth time, they usually sign the forms."

The Counseling Session

Those Bedouin who were instructed, signed the informed consent, provided blood for DNA testing and came to consider a potential engagement, were expected to seek genetic counseling. What follows is a synopsis of a typical counseling encounter. Each encounter is a demonstration of the program's rationale in action, but there is always more than meets the eye in this interaction. The certified counselors speak in Hebrew and know little Arabic. All Bedouin men can speak "practical" Hebrew, but it is not certain whether they understand the more complicated lingo of the counselors. Bedouin women often do not understand Hebrew. The presence of an interpreter (a non-certified Arabic-speaking counselor) is therefore mandatory in such sessions. The public and official character of the encounter, as perceived by the Bedouin, makes it difficult for them (especially for women accompanied by men) to speak out their minds, discussing misunderstandings or asking for explanations. Breaches in communication, pauses and silences, are therefore an inseparable part of the counseling encounter with the Bedouin.

The counseling encounter I describe was conducted with a young Bedouin man who came with another young Bedouin (his cousin, as I later found out), but entered the office of the counselors alone. He was 45 minutes late, but the counselor told me such a delay was quite common and expected with Bedouin counselees. The counselor first introduced me to the counselee and asked for his consent to my presence during the session. He agreed and she asked him for his full name. The session had thus formally begun. It was conducted by the counselor, in Hebrew, except for some Arabic translation.

Counselor: "Is there any deaf person in your family"?

Counselee: "No. I have six healthy brothers and sisters."

Counselor: "Did your father marry a relative, a cousin perhaps?"

Counselee: "No, my mother is not from the family."

At this point the counselor inquired the counselee for about five minutes regarding his, and his partner's, first- and second-degree relatives and whether any of them were deaf. There were hearing-impaired relatives in the family of the counselee's mother. Having found that the partners' parents were related (the fathers were cousins) the counselor told the counselee: "you are practically almost brother and sister!" The counselee was then asked if he brought with him the informed consent of his mate, granting him the right to be counseled in her absence. He took out a letter that was written by one of the community-outreach genetic counselors, where the mate and her mother added their signatures. The counselors looked up the mate's ID. This caused a little havoc since the mate, who was younger than 18, was listed with her mother's ID number.

The counselor then asked: "Do you know about the risk involved in consanguinity?"

The counselee did not answer and the Arabic-speaking counselor who was sitting in the office provided a translation in Arabic, using the local word for consanguinity and asking the counselee whether he understood that children born in marriages that are "made in the family" have a greater risk to be affected by genetic diseases. The counselee said he understood this and the counselor took the lead again.

Counselor: "Are there any other inherited diseases in your family besides deafness?"

Counselee: "Yes, many have a heart disease."

Counselor: "Is it a disease you can die from in young age?"

Counselee: "No. It appears only when they're old."

Counselor: "One more question and then we'll tell you the results. Concerning deafness—do you worry about having deaf children?"

Counselee: "I wouldn't want to have deaf children."

Counselor: "And that's why it's important for you to know the results. But, you must understand that the results I am about to give you are only about deafness. We checked your compatibility only for deafness. Nothing else. When two cousins marry, their children might be affected by lots of diseases. We didn't check these other things, just deafness. According to the test we did, there is almost 100% certainty that you will not have deaf children. Do you understand? You and your mate fit in terms of deafness."

Counselee: "I understand."

Counselor: "but, as cousins you have a lot of common genetic material. If something is wrong with this genetic material, there's a big chance it would be wrong in both of you."

At this point the counselor stopped and asked the counselee if he had any questions. The counselee nodded his head for "No." The session had ended.

The counseling session is interesting for what is missing from the encounter. The public format of the counseling session leaves little elbowroom for explicit negotiation. The result is a separation between the public discourse of counseling and the private realms of attitudes and decision-making. Bedouin counselees generally did not bring their agendas to counseling and did not share them with counselors. This is not a unique phenomenon, of course. It brings to mind other works on the mismatch between patients' and doctors' agendas. Previous studies on interactions with general medical practitioners have shown that only a minority of patients voiced their agendas in consultation (Barry et al., 2000; Stimson and Webb, 1975; Mishler, 1984). Agenda items most commonly voiced were symptoms and requests for diagnoses and prescriptions. The most common unvoiced agenda items were: worries about possible diagnosis and what the future holds; patients' ideas about what is wrong; side effects; not wanting a prescription; and information relating to social context. Agenda items that were not raised in the consultation often led to specific problem outcomes (for example, major misunderstandings), unwanted prescriptions, non-use of prescriptions, and non-adherence to treatment.

The Bedouin Agenda

In an in-depth interview I conducted with Ā'ref (pseudonym), the young Bedouin whose counseling encounter was described above, he said that about five months ago he had begun to think of marrying a cousin of his. Ā'ref said that during this time his family received at-home instruction followed by blood drawing. Ā'ref described his motivation in the following manner:

> "Only now, my involvement [with the girl] became serious and I figured, since I'm probably a carrier and so is she, we will probably test as incompatible. If it were like this I would have used the result in order to cancel everything."

It transpired that Ā'ref experienced pressure from his family, especially from his mother, to make the girl his fiancée. He did not think this was "the right girl" for him and wanted to pull out. According to Ā'ref,

> "This is not a prearranged match, but after I mentioned the girl's name everyone in my family became excited. During the whole year they had already been nudging me why I don't marry. Everyone in my family was already married when they were my age. I got cold feet. In the last month I was thinking about canceling the whole thing. I want to marry once and to have the marriage last for my entire life. I don't want to take a second wife. I will be satisfied with having three or four children. That's enough, as long as they're healthy. I am still young and can bring my wife from outside the clan. I am still young and with plenty of options, despite what my family says."

Ā'ref's story demonstrates an agenda that is different from the program's rationale. While the program intended to encourage marriages between "compatible" mates, the fact that Ā'ref and his mate tested as "compatible" was for him disappointing. Ā'ref wanted to use the counseling for his own purposes. Note that a level of agreement existed between the health aspects of the program and Ā'ref's considerations of susceptibility ("I'm probably a carrier and so is she"; "I will be satisfied with having three or four children [——] as long as they're healthy"). Ā'ref's agenda diverted from the traditional pattern, as demonstrated by the high fertility rates of Bedouin women and the high prevalence of polygyny among the Bedouin — parameters which reflect patterns of fertility behavior considered typical of initial phases of modernization in developing countries (Azaiza, 1996). However, these considerations were secondary in Ā'ref's case. The primary consideration, in his agenda, was his wish to extricate himself from an arranged marriage. Even when he and the girl were found to be compatible, he refused to continue with the match, and the marriage did not take place eventually.

Ā'ref's agenda was not unique. This finding is based on interviews with other Bedouin counselees. In another case, a young Bedouin man called Ahmed (pseudonym) called up the counselor to schedule a meeting. The community-outreach assistant, who knew about the case, arranged for me an interview with Ahmed's older brother, Yaaser (pseudonym) who became head of the family following the death of their father a few years ago. According to my contact person, I would be able to understand this case from Yaaser, because he was "the brain" behind Ahmed's call. Yaaser told me that he was not satisfied with Ahmed's interest in a certain Bedouin girl. He said that according to his calculations, both of them had to be carriers. His idea was that if they take the test, the result would be incompatibility. Like Ā'ref, he planned to use the counseling as a reason for canceling the match.

In another case where the option of counseling was used, a young Bedouin man by the (fictive) name of Abdallah came with his prospective father-in-law (Hussein) for *individual* counseling. Abdallah was informed that he was not a carrier, and his marriage (with Hussein's daughter) took place about a month later. In an interview conducted with Hussein (pseudonym), he explained to me that Abdallah was willing to take the individual test first. The agreement between them was that if Abdallah were not a carrier, than the marriage with Hussein's daughter would take place. If Abdallah were a carrier, then "they would see what to do." The implication was probably that Hussein's daughter would take the test. However this was not said out loud and I was left wondering whether Hussein would actually let his daughter take the test if it would come to that. When asked why he wouldn't start by testing his daughter, he said that she was "too young for that" (this case was also discussed under the section "researching and intervening").

Yet another case involved a Bedouin man who was married to two women. His first wife was healthy while the second wife was hearing-impaired. The man approached the community-outreach counselor and inquired whether he and the second woman could take the test (of carrier matching). He explained that "we are not really married and she can sometimes hear" (interview with community-outreach counselor). In a meeting of the health professionals and counselors it was agreed that the Bedouin man "was being manipulative" and actually wanted to receive a free-of-charge answer regarding his own carrier status. One of the health professionals expressed his concern that married Bedouin men will use the program as a way to screen their wives and/or prospective brides (another case of potential "wife-screening" was described in the context of the instruction session). The dilemma remained unresolved since it was pointed out that simply rejecting the man's request for testing would be to jeopardize his autonomy. One of the health professionals suggested that if a married couple came for carrier matching, the counselor should offer them, free of charge, only information concerning their risk for having an affected child. If the man insisted on receiving an individual answer, he should be told that such an answer would cost 100 USD per each person. Another health professional inquired: "Is this legal?" Nobody in the meeting knew for sure. One of the counselors said: "Perhaps we can tell him his personal carrier status but add that in each new match he must come again to test with the bride." The whole debate reflected the professionals' concern with polygyny and the potential stigmatization of the wife. At the end of the day, this Bedouin man did not show up for testing and counseling. Rather than being solved, the dilemma was merely suspended.

Another counseling session I witnessed, in contrast, conformed to the rationale of the program. It was conducted with a young Bedouin man, his intended fiancée and her father. The young man had a sister with a hearing impairment. The father of the intended fiancée was his second cousin. The counselor told the couple that they were "genetically compatible." In interviews I later conducted separately with both sides, their understanding of the counseling was quite in line with the professional message. When I asked the young man, for example, how he understood the meaning of "compatibility," he answered: "It means that we are not going to have affected babies." He also mentioned that it was a pity that the program did not test for other diseases except deafness, and that he would have taken these tests had they been available. The couple then proceeded to marry as planned. In this case the utilization of genetic counseling conformed to the intended design of the program.

Attitudes of Bedouin Women

So far, I have focused on the attitudes of Bedouin men. By bringing in the agendas of these men, the study shows that medicalization is not a dichotomous process that engenders either compliance or resistance. Rather, the process of medicalization can entail a multiplicity of non-compliant utilization strategies. Like any medical encounter, counseling does not occur in a vacuum. When used, it always becomes entangled in people's lives, and their interests and constraints shape its outcomes.

While personal agendas remained behind the scene, the mismatch between local norms and medical expectations had an explicit aspect in counseling. The model behind carrier matching is a symmetrical dyad—the two mates being perceived (according to Mendelian heredity and Western ethics) as genetically and socially equal. In most of the counseling sessions, however, only the Bedouin man appeared before the counselors, equipped with the signed consent of the girl's father. The counselors, who expected to see both sides, were initially surprised to see just the man appearing before them. For the Bedouin, this expectation challenged the traditional asymmetry of patriarchal status relations.

The emerging pattern of utilization reflected men's attitudes more than women's. In order to understand the attitudes of Bedouin women in regard to the program, a female research assistant conducted semi-structured interviews in Arabic with 28 women (see details in the methodological section). Three main topics were covered in the interviews: etiology and heredity, carrier matching, and abortion. Below are representative excerpts relating to these themes.

Etiology and Heredity

> "Some women have a strong eye. This ability becomes stronger during pregnancy. For example, if I'm pregnant and I watch the liver of a lamb while it is being slaughtered. I feel like eating the liver, but I don't. At that moment I scratch my body with my hand. It means there will be a mark in the body of my fetus, in the same spot where I scratched. When I give birth, my child's body will show that thing which I strongly felt for. If a pregnant woman looks at a deaf child, and she feels strongly about it, deafness will then pass to her fetus, and this is why more deaf children are born. It happens a lot in our family."

> "A woman can transform the image in front of her into her body. I stayed at home during all my pregnancies for that reason. In addition, I don't watch TV programs of a kind that I shouldn't transform into my body unhealthy images."

The embodiment of images into the fetal body through the 'strong eye' of pregnant women is an interesting anthropological phenomenon. In the psychoanalytical tradition, embodiment is a phenomenon that projects some sort of unconscious fixations onto the body. There are, for example, numerous psychoanalytical studies of the embodiment of long-term psychological effects of incest by victims (Young, 1992). Such studies focus on the trauma and dissociation linked with sexual abuse in terms of the problem of embodiment.

Anthropologists, in contrast, have focused on the presumably universal cultural perception of the ambiguity of women's body boundaries during birth and menstruation (Comaroff, 1992). In our case, the pregnant mother is thought to project inside her body a powerful image seen by her in the outside world, thus inscribing a physical equivalent of this image onto her fetus' body. This explanation joins other indigenous accounts of the natural (rather than personal) power of a pregnant woman to determine the traits of her fetus as a result of strong and particularly unfulfilled desires she experiences (Sacks, 1997; Hand, 1980). This phenomenon is generally called *hulf* (literally to give birth to something different) by the Bedouin, and is broadly used to explain differences in appearance between a child and its parents. For example, a Bedouin may explain the birth of light-skinned child to dark-skinned parents by saying that they had neighbors with light-skinned children who used to play under the supervision of the pregnant mother. This phenomenon represents an active ability of women but does not assume good or bad intention (as in the case of the 'evil eye,' another accepted belief among the Bedouin). In the context of congenital hearing loss, the mother could explain that she was pre-occupied by the conduct, looks or behavior of a deaf person. For example, a pregnant woman could be said to bring deafness onto her fetus by having "looked too long at two deaf people communicating through sign language, which she didn't understand." Or, maybe she "looked at someone who is deaf but also good-looking, and felt compassion and sadness that the person doesn't hear" (see Kisch, 2000: 190–91). Similar accounts were available in regard to the etiology of thalassemia. In this case, the trait that was emphasized in the stories was "weak blood."

In addition, women spoke in a different way than men about the heredity of the disease. For example:

> "We knew all along that it is men who are the cause of it. Men plant the seed in the soil. Men give the seed. You reap what you sow."

Many women voiced this opinion in reply to the standard question regarding stepwise testing ("what do you think about the following system: someone does the test for himself. If he has the gene for the disease, then he should ask his bride to test, too. If he doesn't have the gene, then it doesn't matter whom he marries. What do you think about such a system?"). In contrast, most men answered that while stepwise testing was a valid option, it stigmatized women. Therefore this option was less desirable in the Bedouin context. In addition, many women believed that stepwise testing was bad because it did not prevent the births of carriers. This criticism could be extended to integrative disclosure:

> "If someone took the test for himself and knows that he doesn't have the gene for the disease, he cannot pick up any woman he likes without the test. This would not be right. Such a man thinks only about himself, and he doesn't think about his children. Maybe the woman he marries has the gene and then their children will get it from her."

The prevalence of this reply among Bedouin women appears to reflect a greater concern for the quality (rather than quantity) of progeny. "Integrative disclosure" does not discourage the marriage of a carrier and a non-carrier. Therefore the children of a couple that is "genetically compatible" may indeed be carriers.

The women's opinion that a child's important traits are inherited from the father could be seen as a counter-argument to an alternative narrative, voiced by some of the men, that blamed the origin of deafness on a "foreigner" woman who was married to one of the clan's ancestors. These alternative and gendered accounts were hybrid forms of discourse, employing "scientific" semantics within a local cultural syntax. "Blood," for example, represented for many community members a symbol of monogenetic, gender-specific inheritance (see also Kisch, 2000: 183–86). The common image of the father who 'plants the seed' and the mother as providing 'the soil' supports the view of male-specific or patrilineal heredity (see also Delaney, 1991; Fedida, 1984). Indeed, the Bedouin worldview considers blood ties to be primarily agnatic or patrilineal (Kressel, 1992), while female blood ties are regarded as weaker (Abu-Lughod, 1986). The Arabic word for heredity (*waratha*) comes from the same semantic root as inheritance.

Carrier Matching

> "Let me give you an example. Hussein's daughter married with El-Ouda and she has no deaf children. Her sister married Abdul and they did have deaf children [all names have been changed]. You can't tell in advance. It is better to go and take the test. You tell us because you see the answer in the blood. If a girl does not match someone, she can still match another, not necessarily the one who wanted her in the first place. This is how you explained it to us, isn't it? If you don't marry this person you can still marry another. If that girl doesn't match, maybe her sister will. These things have happened."

To begin with, many women regarded consanguinity as a positive situation that provides social protection. When Bedouin men or health professionals mentioned that consanguinity was a "good thing for women," this could probably be interpreted as paternalism. I therefore emphasize that this argument was also heard from many Bedouin women. Some women spoke about consanguinity as a "safety net" (see parallel references in Darr's 1990: 284–86 study of British Pakistanis). Similar positive references to consanguinity also characterized the Bedouin female respondents in another ethnographic study:

> "And if I marry this man [a Bedouin from South Hevron, about 100 km from the Negev and not related to her family], who will I be there, how will I be treated? Where will I go when there are problems? Here we know each other, and if I have problems, I am surrounded by family. If my husband treats me rudely, I can go to my neighbor, my sister. If he decides that my daughter has to stop going to school—I will raise hell. I will go to everyone and not let it happen—whether she's hearing or deaf!" (Kisch, 2000: 206, interview with a Bedouin female respondent].

Carrier matching was therefore positively considered within the framework of consanguinity. In that sense the women's interpretation was closer to the program's message of "healthy consanguinity," whereas some of the men interpreted the message as encouraging out-marriage. These different "interpretive norms" reflect a situation in which the clan's status is affirmed by giving the least number of daughters in exogamy relative to the larger number of "stranger" or agnatic outsider brides (*gharība*) brought into the family. I do not have actual data on the number of "stranger" brides brought into the clan as compared to the number of daughters given in exogamy during the period of the research. However, in interviews with clan members it was obvious for men and women that bringing in "stranger" brides was quite acceptable for Bedouin men, whereas Bedouin women were expected to be taken for brides by their cousins (see also Kressel, 1980: 20–21).

There is a possible linkage between women's positive view of consanguinity and the various alternative accounts for heredity and etiology that were voiced by them. These explanations may have used essential symbols of "blood" and "genes," but in a way that was essentially discursive, manipulating these symbols according to the social, micro-political and gendered interests of speakers. The multiplicity of alternative explanations (voiced by women as well as men) to the biomedical model of hereditary diseases may have contributed to the low uptake of genetic services by the Bedouin. Some respondents claimed that the genetic explanation was not the only one, and that it was very difficult to track with precision all the reasons behind hereditary diseases and congenital disorders. Such a stance implied that there was no place for a drastic intervention such as premarital carrier matching through genetic testing.

The alternative etiological accounts voiced by Bedouin men and women—despite their evident variability—shared a common denominator. All of them shifted the "blame" from *consanguinity* to other sources. None of these explanations was presented as parsimonious. According to such explanations, either the 'blood' or 'seed' of the father caused the disease, or the 'strong eye' (or breast milk) of the mother—but evidently *not* the marriage of cousins, as claimed by health professionals. Both Bedouin men and women subscribed to these explanations and could use them as a way of putting the blame on the opposite sex. The higher prevalence of such explanations among women is conventionally explained by their relatively lower education. Another interesting explanation focuses on women's greater dependence on in-group match making. Women are passively "taken in marriage" while men actively "take brides." However, many women regarded consanguinity as a safety net in a society that is heavily dominated by men. By focusing on the role of either the father or the mother in regard to heredity, consanguinity was purged, and its practice could thus continue, with or without medical interventions such as carrier matching.

Abortion

> "I do what the doctor decides. If the doctor tells me to do an abortion, I'll do it. We have suffered enough in our lives. I got married when I was 15. Today I have 11 children. Look at me, how I look, I don't care about religion. The main thing is my health and my children's health. I don't remember how my children grew up. Look at them, every year I gave birth to another one. I'm pregnant now with another one. Look at me, isn't it enough that we have to go through this much. To have a crippled or deaf child on top of it—I wouldn't accept such a thing, if it were up to me."

> "Sure I'll abort if the fetus is sick. What am I, crazy? I would do abortion even if I was five, six, seven months pregnant. Look at me now, I'm pregnant and can hardly move. I have grown-up daughters who are a great help. Without them I would have collapsed. Imagine that on top of that I will have a sick child. It can't be imagined."

> "Why suffer all your life when you can select a better option from the start. Nobody will come to help me if—God forbid—I'll have a sick child. I will be angry and bitter all my life and the child will suffer from the disease all his life. I have my own free will to decide what is good and what is bad in such moments. In such moments I do not think about Islam. I have seen enough suffering with my child."

Although some Bedouin men also said they would agree to abortion due to hearing loss or other genetic diseases, they were in the minority. The prevalence of this view among women was much more salient. Of the 28 women who were interviewed, 16 (57%) agreed that abortion was a good idea in cases of genetic diseases (including hearing loss). The narrative of care and suffering with which many of the women framed their pro-abortion attitude was not typical of men. It was arguably the result of a gendered division of labor in which women take all the responsibility for caring for children (Abu-Lughod, 1986). Men, however, make decisions regarding family planning. In Bedouin society, a large number of children traditionally represented the family's "human resource" and was hence encouraged. This strategy was aptly termed "competitive breeding" by Kressel (1992). Many of the younger Bedouin generation were critical of this attitude in interviews. They blamed it for preferring quantity to quality and underplaying the health of progeny. Note also the words of Ā'ref, the young Bedouin man mentioned earlier in the context of the counseling session, who claimed: "I want to marry once and to have the marriage last for my entire life. I don't want to take a second wife. I will be satisfied with having three or four children. That's enough, as long as they're healthy." Ā'ref's agenda was actually quite typical of the younger, more educated Bedouin generation. However, it has not yet changed the traditional pattern. It appears that "competitive breeding," just like family planning decisions in general, was constituted as part of men's (rather than women's) traditional agenda.

In a study that focused on the use of prenatal screening among Negev Bedouin women (Lewando-Hundt et al., 2001), it was found that Bedouin women understand that consanguinity can lead to the birth of impaired children. The women interviewed for that study also made frequent references to God's will (*kull ishee min Allah*) and to the role of chance (*naseeb*). These local beliefs could indeed explain the low uptake of prenatal tests by Negev Bedouin women in general. Almost all the Bedouin women who attended the clinics for prenatal care had at least one ultrasound at some point during pregnancy. However, uptake of further screening tests for congenital malformations and hereditary diseases was much lower. Only a few of those referred actually undertook the tests. Neither consanguinity, maternal age nor maternal or paternal education were associated with the uptake of tests. The only strong and significant predictor of test uptake was the death of a previous child. Mothers who had lost a child were more likely to undergo fetal screening.

In interviews held by Lewando-Hundt et al. (2001) in the homes of 16 Bedouin mothers, respondents were much more critical of the reliability of prenatal screening tests (including ultrasound, the triple test, and amniocentesis) than the Bedouin women interviewed for this study. These Bedouin mothers argued that both the consequences of consanguinity and the tests are uncertain in their outcomes, and frequently cited "false alarm" stories as a way of illustrating how wrong the results of screening may be. According to the interpretation offered by Lewando-Hundt et al (2001), the low uptake of prenatal screening tests by these Bedouin women represents 'resistance.' These women are described by the researchers as making rational choices regarding the appropriate level of surveillance of their bodies, as do modern women in Japan and the USA (Lock, 1998; Rapp, 1998).

In this study, in contrast, women appear (at least in personal interviews) as being pro-abortion and interested in using genetic tests. No criticism regarding the reliability of tests was voiced. However, this study also shows that amniocentesis is conducted (or, as is more often the case, avoided) according to men's agendas. Obviously, the major reason for the low uptake of amniocentesis is the religious ban on abortion. In addition, it should be recalled that the Bedouin women interviewed for this study were instructed about human genetics and genetic testing, while the women interviewed by Lewando-Hundt et al. (2001) were not. Susceptibility, shown by Levando-Hundt et al. (2001) to be the only strong and significant predictor of test uptake, was also relevant to the Bedouin women studied here, all of whom were members of an at-risk population where the prevalence of genetic diseases was particularly high.

Thalassemia did not trigger the same array of alternative explanations as NSRD. Rather, the genetic explanation provided in the instruction was regarded by the majority of Bedouin respondents as "more accurate." The relatively higher socio-economic status and level of education of community members, as well as the severity of the disease, could be the main reasons for this situation. Consequently, the at-risk population was also willing to try out the carrier matching system proposed by the program. Pro-abortion attitudes were also common. In private interviews some of the newly wed younger Bedouin with a family history of thalassemia said they did the early prenatal genetic test (CVS) on their initiative and without telling their parents. They had to go for the purpose of CVS to a distant hospital in Tel-Aviv. This also attests to their motivation and high level of medical awareness—something that was not apparent in the context of congenital hearing loss.

Chapter 5

Cross-Cultural Genetics Education: Between Acculturation and Ambivalence

Providing multicultural genetics education is a major challenge to the profession of genetic counseling. Traditional counseling has been predominantly designed for Euro-Americans, and the majority of genetic counselors are not members of ethnically diverse groups (Weil, 2000). One of the goals of this study was to investigate the efficacy of multicultural genetics education in a traditional non-western society. About half of the Bedouin population is under the age of 14 years old. This means that school education can provide a tremendous catalyst for social change. In this chapter I focus on the attitudes of Bedouin adolescents, who were taught the new genetics curriculum, and their teachers.

Data were collected using a two-part self-report questionnaire consisting of 14 items. The first part inquired about possibly relevant background variables such as age, education, gender, geographic origin (in the case of teachers) and genetic diseases in the family, and assessed the knowledge of basic genetic information. The second part of the questionnaire asked about attitudes towards genetic testing and reproductive decisions. The quantitative measurement of the questionnaire was complemented by semi-structured discussions in focus groups.

Questions assessing knowledge of and attitudes towards genetic testing were confirmed through a pilot study involving six genetic counselors who commented on the validity of the questionnaire. In a manner parallel to genetics education programs, the questionnaire sought to define the fewest, simplest pieces of information that should be included. All counselors agreed, for example, that the recessive mode of inheritance is the single most important message to introduce, because it shows that anyone may be a carrier without having an affected individual in the family (i.e., genetics involves us all), and it prepares students for later offers of screening. For this reason the knowledge section focused on the subject of recessive inheritance.

During 1999–2001 meetings were conducted with five groups of pupils and seven groups of teachers. These groups represented Bedouin schools in cities as well as in "unrecognized" areas. Groups of pupils had eight participants on average, consisting of male and female 9th graders. The five groups (n=40) represented five different schools, where pupils studied the same curriculum in human genetics prior to the meetings. Meetings lasted about three hours and were coordinated in Arabic by one of the research assistants. The seven groups of teachers (n= 61) were recruited from the same schools as well as from other schools in the area. The meetings with teachers lasted about three hours and were conducted in one of the school's rooms. The same questionnaire was administered to the pupils and the teachers.

Knowledge of Basic Genetic Information

The first part of the questionnaire assessed the efficacy of cross-cultural education regarding genetics. The first table summarizes the results of the teachers and the schoolchildren (see Table 4).

Questionnaire items were selected based on the counselors' notion of what factual information was essential in order to make an informed use of pre-marital genetic counseling. Teachers' average knowledge index was 80.75 (representing the average percent of correct answers in all eight questions). Although relatively high, such a "score" was disappointing since those teachers were trained and instructed to perform the role of socialization agents. Schoolchildren's average knowledge index (64.43) was even lower. The difference between males and females in terms of knowledge was insignificant. A correlation was found between the score of teachers and pupils in specific questions, i.e., questions in which a high percent of teachers knew the correct answer were also those in which a (relatively) high percent of pupils knew the correct answer. The knowledge index of those teachers and pupils who studied the genetics curriculum was compared to the knowledge index of those who did not, and the latter was found to be significantly lower.

Table 4. Frequency of Correct Results for Teachers and Pupils

Question	Pupils	Teachers
1. A carrier of recessive disease does not suffer from that disease.	T 38.5%	78%
2. A carrier of recessive disease does not develop it later in life.	T 40%	70%
3. If a healthy child is born to carriers, probably all their children will be healthy too.	F 80%	93%
4. Parents who are both carriers of recessive disease have 25% risk at each pregnancy of having an affected child.	T 70%	87%
5. Parents who are carriers of recessive disease have 50% risk at each pregnancy of having an affected child.	F 51%	58%
6. Consanguinity increases the prevalence of recessive disease.	T 90%	98%
7. There are hereditary diseases that can be transmitted through breast-feeding.	F 59%	80%
8. A child receives genetic traits from his/her: (a) father, (b) mother, (c) God, (d) equally from his father and mother.	(d) 87%	82%

Results in percents, for teachers (n=61) and pupils (n=40).
T = True, F = False.
Question 8, unlike the other questions, is multiple choice.

Attitudes towards Genetic Counseling

Two indexes were constructed for the purpose of analyzing attitudes towards genetic counseling. The first denoted positive-negative attitudes on a range of 1 to 9 (1 = decidedly negative, 9 = decidedly positive). The second index denoted an alternative attitude that relayed the responsibility for decisions to one's family. The "family dependent" attitude was on a range of 0 (min.) to 5 (max.). Scores contributing to the two indexes were mutually exclusive, since the response of one subject to one question could only contribute to one or the other index, not to both. In both cases, indexes were constructed from relevant items within the multiple-choice questions in the second part of the questionnaire. These questions covered topics that were germane to genetic counseling and reproductive descisions, such as: the cost and benefit of premarital and prenatal diagnosis, the use of genetic compatibility testing for marital decisions, the meaning of consanguinity, and general attitudes towards genetic testing. For example, we asked the respondents whether they would

Table 5. Hypothetical Decisions of Teachers and Schoolchildren about Personal Use of Premarital Genetic Testing

	Teachers	Schoolchildren	
		Females (n=22)	Males (n=18)
1. I would certainly not ask for premarital diagnosis.	0	0	12
2. I would probably not ask for premarital diagnosis.	0	6	12
3. I would probably ask for premarital diagnosis.	20	5	47
4. I would certainly ask for premarital diagnosis.	77	64	12
5. I would ask for premarital diagnosis if it were up to me, but my family would object.	0	5	12
6. I would consult my family and decide accordingly.	3	23	6

teachers (n=61), schoolchildren (n=40).
All numbers are in percents.

use premarital diagnosis, provided that there was a genetic test for a disease that supposedly ran in their family (Table 5).

Articles 1–4 in Table 2 were counted in the negative-positive index (article 1 and 2 represent a negative attitude, while 3 and 4 represent a positive attitude). Articles 5 and 6 in Table 2 were counted in the 'family dependent' index. The same question was repeated in regard to hypothetical decisions about recommending pre-marital genetic testing to progeny. 95% of the teachers and 89% of the schoolchildren (81% males, 95% females) replied positively to this question. This high percentage could reflect the future reduction of inter-generational conflict.

Based on the questions, the following attitudes were found (Table 6).

Table 6. General Attitudes towards Genetic Testing

	Teachers	Schoolchildren		Range
		M	F	
Positive–Negative	7.65	6.65	7.0	1 (negative)–9 (positive)
Family dependent	0.16	0.44	0.68	0 (min.)–5 (max.)

teachers (n=61), schoolchildren: male (n=22), female (n=18).

Table 6 shows that in general, teachers were more positive about genetic counseling (7.65 on a scale of 1–9). Male and female schoolchildren were also positive, although to a slightly less degree (6.65 and 7 on a scale of 1–9). The hypothesis was that teachers' better familiarity with genetics education resulted in a more positive attitude towards the program. In terms of the Health Belief Model, teachers have more knowledge about genetics, thus being more positive about genetic counseling. The hypothesis regarding the effect of an inter-generational conflict (the negative attitude of the more traditional parents towards genetic counseling) was not validated by the second index. "Family dependence" was found to be very low (near minimum) in the attitudes of teachers as well as schoolchildren.

Correlation between Knowledge and Attitudes

Pearson correlation was used to examine the relationship between knowledge of genetics (represented by the knowledge index) and attitudes towards genetic counseling among teachers and schoolchildren. A positive correlation ($r=0.38$, $p=0.01$) between knowledge of genetics and a positive attitude towards genetic testing was found. Distribution analysis showed that more than half of the teachers (64%) who had a high knowledge index (75–100), were also positive towards the program (measured by an attitude index in the range of 7–9). In contrast, only 7% of the teachers who had a low knowledge index were positive toward the program. The majority of pupils (60%), who were characterized by a medium knowledge index (a range of 51–75), also had a positive stance towards the program, measured by an attitude index in the range of 7–9. In contrast, only 8% of the pupils who had a low knowledge index were positive toward the program.

Susceptibility, Knowledge and Attitudes

The health belief model predicts that susceptibility is a major factor in the construction of health beliefs. We asked the respondents whether they have relatives with a genetic disease. 33% of the pupils and 29% of the teachers reported having family members (in various kinship levels) who were affected by a genetic disease. Susceptibility was found to correlate with knowledge of genetics across all the respondents ($rs= .31$, $p<.05$). For example, schoolchildren who were not susceptible had an average knowledge index of 61, while schoolchildren who had an affected brother or sister (first-level kinship designating "highest" susceptibility) had an average knowledge index of 71. Similarly, teachers who were not susceptible had an average knowledge index of 79, while teachers who had an affected brother or sister had an average knowledge index of 86. The correlation between susceptibility and attitude was not significant. Schoolchildren who were not susceptible had a 6.9 score on the negative-positive attitude scale, while schoolchildren who were susceptible scored 7 on that scale. There was no significant difference between male and female schoolchildren in regard to the effect of susceptibility. It is probable that since all pupils were exposed to the same genetics education, this became the major factor behind their positive knowledge, thus overshadowing the possible differentiating effect of susceptibility.

Questionnaires have their limitations in eliciting beliefs and attitudes, mainly due to their artificial, standard framework which lacks subjective orientation and may create misunderstandings due to language and communication barriers. Indeed, somewhat different responses were obtained in the group discussions conducted with the same respondents who answered the questionnaires. These two sources of information (questionnaires and group discussions) were juxtaposed in order to increase the validity of interpretation.

A major finding was that premarital genetic testing was regarded positively by the majority of respondents. Furthermore, the respondents' knowledge of genetics and positive attitude towards genetic counseling, which were both significantly raised by genetics education, were also positively correlated ($r=.38$, $p=.01$). The major difference between teachers and pupils was the relatively lower knowledge index of pupils and their relatively lower degree of positive attitude. It was actually expected that pupils' attitudes would be even less positive, following ambivalent remarks voiced by them in the context of group discussions. Such ambivalence would have been in line with the complex situation of Bedouin adolescents as being "between and betwixt" modern genetics education and traditional Bedouin culture. Interestingly, family dependence—a local cultural factor that could interfere with genetically-informed individual attitudes—was shown to be of minimal importance for pupils. This may also suggest that local cultural norms in the spheres of religion and culture are not perceived as *family*-dependent, having been internalized as the responsibility of the individual.

Group discussions with the same respondents showed that the effect of susceptibility (to familial genetic disorders) may be compromised by the traditional importance of and lack of alternatives to consanguinity, as well as by the sense of susceptibility to the stigma associated with positive carrier status. Such stigma was particularly apparent in the context of women, and many of the respondents (both teachers and pupils) commented that if a woman were found to be a carrier, this would make it difficult for her to get married as a first wife. Furthermore, respondents commented that individual disclosure would not keep the carrier status confidential, since "information like this travels fast in our community." Many of the male respondents said that in case of individual disclosure, they would insist on asking the girl's father whether she was a carrier before considering the option of marriage. Hence, individual carrier status (particularly of women) would become part of the premarital negotiation phase. It therefore appears that the intervention program was correct in its emphasis on carrier matching as a means for reducing stigmatization.

Group discussions also revealed that, in the eyes of respondents, one of the program's advantages was the availability of specific genetic tests. In a study of premarital genetic counseling to Jewish consanguineous couples in Israel, the majority (72%) proceeded with their plans and married their relatives, and many (86%) expressed disappointment at not being offered specific genetic tests (Shiloh et al., 1995). Premarital counseling is perceived by counselees as being too general when not involving specific genetic tests, a fact that should be born in mind before initiating community-based multicultural genetic education as well as counseling.

Concepts of genetic heredity and probability may also be mis- or partially understood in the context of indigenous beliefs and experiences. A study of parental responses to genetic disease in Saudi Arabia reported that indigenous explanations focused on asymmetrical inheritance of hereditary diseases, particularly through the mother (Panter-Brick, 1991). In group discussions, pupils said they heard about local beliefs that link congenital diseases and fetal deformations to "the strong eye" (see also Abu-Rabi'a 1983, 1999) of pregnant women, but many said these beliefs were "irrational." Nevertheless, the ubiquity of such beliefs may be one of the factors behind the low knowledge index of the pupils. About 40% of the pupils, as we saw, thought that there are hereditary diseases that can be transmitted through breast-feeding, and 60% of them thought that a carrier of a recessive disease can suffer from that disease.

Finally, we also have to consider the program as an interface between the dominant Jewish medical establishment and an ethnic minority—the Bedouin. Some pupils said in group discussions that elders in their family were prejudiced against the program, seeing it as an Israeli-Jewish attempt to reduce the Bedouin birth rate. These pupils commented, however, that in their opinion such interpretations represented insufficient medical and genetic understanding. Schoolchildren are therefore an appropriate study group for getting more insight into community opinions about genetic education, screening and counseling. When applying cross-cultural genetics education, teachers and professionals should be aware that they are entering a sensitive zone of prejudice and preconceptions and that their teachings could in fact fuel inter-generational conflict. Further research is needed, as these schoolchildren grow up and plan to get married, on their actual uptake of genetic testing—premarital and prenatal—and how it is used for reproductive decisions.

Chapter 6

Questions of Reception

In its attempt to change traditional patterns of attitudes and behavior, the experimental program for carrier matching included the implementation of at-home educational sessions, genetics education at school, and community-outreach genetics referral service provided in Mother and Child Clinics. These activities were conducted in addition to the conventional screening and counseling provided at the medical center. In this chapter I focus on yet another form of communication that was used for promoting carrier matching and genetic counseling in general, namely a filmed documentary drama entitled 'Āysha.' Media technologies such as films are rarely introduced into the curriculum of Bedouin schools. In that sense the production, public relations and utilization of the film 'Āysha' required creativity and dedication.

The 50-minute film 'Āysha' is a documentary drama that demonstrates the pros and cons of match making and genetic testing. Partially funded by the Israeli TV in Arabic, this film was shown on national TV at least twice, and has been repeatedly shown to Bedouin pupils as part of a new curriculum on human genetics and family planning. The film epitomizes the program's rationale by purporting to translate medical terms and thinking into local cultural terms and speak to local customs such as Islamic bans on abortion and agnatic consanguinity. The film serves as a basis for group discussions and activities at school, thus extending the more conventional curriculum based on frontal teaching.

"Āysha": Staging the Drama of Carrier Matching

The documentary drama "Āysha" was produced in 1999 as part of the new curriculum in human genetics intended for Bedouin schools. A narrative analysis of Āysha's scripts is supplemented by observations from discussions of the program's steering committee, which was responsible for the film. During 2001 meetings were conducted with five groups of Bedouin pupils and seven groups of teachers, already described in the context of the questionnaire on knowledge and attitudes (see previous chapter). 'Āysha' was also shown and discussed in the context of these meetings. During 2002, six more meetings with a total of 81 participants were conducted in Bedouin schools with 'Āysha' serving as a focal point for discussion.

The story of 'Āysha,' the film, captures the drama of the whole intervention program. The following quote describes the great expectations felt by health professionals in the context of the film:

> "Shooting the film took about two weeks, but we worked on the script for about a year before it could take place. I went through the script word by word, and changed everything that was potentially deleterious. For example, there is a Bedouin tradition that women are responsible for genetic diseases. There are specific words that imply this, for example when you say that the mother was sick—even if she was only a carrier—and therefore her children are sick too. We were very careful not to use any of these words in order to avoid a stigmatic connotation. It was hard work [...] I know this population. I know what they feel and what their mentality is like. I also belong to the Genetics Institute, and I want to deliver our message. It was a very delicate task—how to deliver our message without hurting the feelings of Bedouin society. You cannot tell them 'don't marry your cousins.' You cannot tell them 'go on and marry your cousins but you're going to have sick children.' You need to find something that is fitting for the 21st century, which says that Bedouin tradition should be left behind. It is a very delicate and important message." [Interview with a Bedouin doctor, member of the program's steering committee.]

The film was produced for instruction purposes. The program's steering committee contracted a director of documentary dramas, who suggested this genre as suitable for the purposes of community engagement. In the director's original conception, the film was to be shot in a Bedouin town and played by "real" Bedouin people (rather than by professional actors). The intention, in postmodern terminology, was to construct a "staged authenticity" (McCannell, 1976a,b) or a "simulation" (Baudrillard, 1983, 1988). After auditioning local youth in a Bedouin village, the shooting was stopped by family members of the Bedouin girl who was selected to play the lead female role (called Āysha). They claimed that the film shamed the family because it involved a staged love affair between the lead female and male actors. Authenticity (community norms) and stage (the film) were therefore indeed mixed, but not in the way expected by the producers. Having re-encountered a similar problem in another Bedouin town, it was decided to move the production to neighboring Jordan. The film was shot in the Jordanian desert with professional Arab actors playing the lead roles and a Jordanian medical doctor playing himself. The script retained the ideological emphasis on a positive message regarding the importance of genetic testing and the reproductive risk inherent in consanguinity. It also maintained the illusion of realistic documentation. Actors were directed to improvise on the basis of the scenario so as to create a more authentic ambiance. At the end of the film, a narrator recounted what happened to the characters, as if they were real people.

The Script and Its Versions

'Āysha' tells the story of an assertive young Bedouin female named Āysha, who is living with her family in a hamlet. All dialogues are in Arabic. The film opens with a conversation between Āysha and her sister, Jamīla. Āysha tells Jamīla about her intended fiancé, Mahmūd (Jamīla's brother). Jamīla replies: "Look at me. I married my cousin according to tradition. Look at my child. Four years old and you can't tell it." We are told that Jamīla's son suffers from an inherited disease. The name and symptoms of the disease are not disclosed. In the following scene, Jamīla, her son, and Āysha are at the Mother and Child clinic. Having heard that Jamīla is pregnant, the nurse tells her: "It is important that you take the tests. The first test is done in week 9–11 and it can tell you if your child is sick. Another test is amniocentesis. Some mistakenly call it the "head fluid" (*mayim tel ras*) test. They put a needle in your stomach, as you can see in the drawing (the nurse shows a schematic drawing of the amniocentesis process to Jamīla). They draw the fluid and send it to the lab. It is a low-risk test. Only one in 200 women miscarries. There are other tests: blood and ultrasound. God willing, your baby will be healthy." Turning to Ā ysha, the nurse asks Jamīla: "Who is that beautiful girl?"
Jamīla: "My sister Āysha. I hope she marries my cousin."
Nurse: "Why? Haven't you learned a lesson? Look at your son. Why are you repeating the same mistake? [To Āysha:] You should take the test intended for people marrying relatives."

This is the first encounter with an agent of socialization (the nurse). The nurse (played by a Bedouin, although most nurses are Jewish-Israelis who speak little Arabic) mentions the early test (CVS, chorionic villus sampling) although this test was not offered at the local medical center at the time of the study, and then considers amniocentesis at length. When talking to Āysha, the nurse mentions the carrier matching premarital test. The nurse thus covers all types of genetic testing, prenatal and premarital, in a very directive manner which is also very impersonal and general, since no family history is taken and there is no mention of the concrete disease and whether a genetic test indeed exists for that disease.

In the following scenes, Āysha asks Jamīla to convince her husband to talk with Mahmūd about taking the test. Āysha then talks with her mother and asks her to convince Āysha's father regarding the necessity of the test. Āysha's mother is very pessimistic in the beginning, saying: "Why are you going to take a test? There's nothing wrong with you." When Āysha insists, her mother says: "Your father will object. What came to Jamīla and her husband, came from God and not from any Doctor. I married your father, my cousin, and we never did any tests. If people will start talking, your father will kill us!"

These scenes portray two important motifs that will later re-emerge as essential dilemmas in the plot. First, it shows the gendered status relations of patriarchal Bedouin society. Āysha cannot approach other men (her intended fiancé and her father) directly. She uses "middle-women" (her mother and Jamīla) to speak on her behalf to their husbands. Second, we witness an intergenerational gap between the young generation (like Āysha, Jamīla and Mahmūd) and the elders, who are the keepers of tradition. At the end of the scene, Āysha's mother unexpectedly changes her mind and says: "Very good. Your father is going away on Thursday, do it then."

The following scene takes place in the medical center. Āysha, Jamīla, and Mahmūd sit in front of a doctor who explains the test to them. The doctor says: "the test is harmless and it's for your own good. You don't want to have a sick child. A sick child is a heavy burden. Visits to hospitals, he will always be sick. All your money will go to medical attention."

Mahmūd: "Does the test reveal if one of us is sick and the other isn't?"

Doctor: "genetic diseases are passed on the genes which are situated on chromosomes. If both the father and mother carry the gene, there is a 25 per cent chance that your child will be sick. Do you understand? It is better for you to take the test, since you are relatives, right?

Jamīla: "We're here because we fear these things."

Doctor: "If you fear that, you should take the test. Then you'll know that it isn't the mother's fault. I stress that both parents are equally responsible. It isn't just the mother's responsibility. You are both responsible so you should both take the test."

During the whole conversation, Āysha does not speak, but keeps sneaking glances at Mahmūd. When they are back at the hospital to receive the test results, the doctor says: "I'm afraid you both carry the gene. You're not sick yourselves."

Mahmūd: "The test is wrong, doctor."
Doctor: "It is a lab test."
Mahmūd: "Wrong, doctor. I don't carry it, I don't know if she carries it. I'm not sick, doctor."
Doctor: "Like I said, you are not sick. You are not sick! You carry the gene. You might pass it to your children, but you are not sick."
Mahmūd: "The test is wrong."
Doctor: "I'm not making this up. This is a lab test. I have a few suggestions. You can get married if you want."
Mahmūd: "Yes, I want to marry her."
Doctor: "I don't forbid it. But she's your cousin, and you must do a test at every pregnancy to discover the disease at an early stage. Without these tests, you're responsible for having sick kids. This is my opinion: Preventive medicine is better than a sea of medication. It's better not to have a sick or retarded child, who'll be a burden. You'll have to spend time and money on doctors, who won't help. There is no complete cure for these illnesses"

The doctor's words illustrate a basic ethical dilemma of genetic counseling, namely nondirectivess. In an international attitude survey administered to genetic counselors (Wertz, 1998), widespread support was expressed for people's right to choose their mates even if these choices increased their risk of having children with a genetic disorder. The majority of counselors in most nations disagreed with the statement that "people who carry a recessive gene should not mate with another carrier of the same recessive gene" (Wertz, 1998: 502). These attitudes represent the 'standard view' of genetic counseling, which consists of universal criteria such as informed consent, nondirectiveness, and autonomy.

The doctor's words and attitude are very directive. Although he "did not forbid" the marriage (which is in itself a surprisingly directive manner of speech), he made clear that in his opinion it would be the parent's responsibility to do a test at every pregnancy and abort an affected fetus. He never used the direct word "abortion," probably because of the religious ban. Yet he repeatedly explained why a sick child is "a burden" for his parents and why "preventive medicine is better than a sea of medication." Note also the doctor's emphasis on the equal responsibility of the parents. As this study has shown, indigenous Bedouin explanations focus on asymmetrical inheritance of genetic diseases through the "strong eye" of the pregnant woman, breast-feeding, or "blood."

According to one of the health professionals who oversaw the film's production, the Jordanian physician's appearance was not planned. The scene was filmed at a local physician's office who, at the last minute, insisted on playing the physician's role, a role which was originally reserved for a Bedouin community-outreach assistant (referred to as Yusuf in the description of the instruction session). As there was no written script, the MD conveyed the message the way he saw fit. Because the film's director (a Jewish-Israeli man) was not fluent in Arabic, Yusuf was probably the only person who actually understood in real time what the MD was saying. "When the film was at the editing phase," the health professional commented, "we made great efforts to edit out messages that we did not think would have occurred in a counseling session in the Genetics Institute, but the scene [with the Jordanian doctor] could not be re-done. We did our best but we were not happy with the final result. Neither were we happy with the performance of the nurse at the Mother and Child Health clinic."

From this point the script focuses on the family drama. At the *shiqq* (the public part of the tent or the house), the men of the family gather to discuss the test results. One of them says, "if she carries the disease, it must come from her mother's side." Another elder comments: "they're unlucky. All things must end. Find a new bride for your son!" The wedding is off and Āysha is ordered not to leave the house any more (not even to school) since she disobeyed her father by going to the doctor without his permission. She refuses to become the second wife of Sāmir, another cousin, who is an old and wealthy man.

Enter Ismā'īl, a friend of Jamīla's husband, who is interested in Āysha. Ismā 'īl speaks about how "the old ways of marrying relatives must change." He tells his friends, "in the days of the prophet, it was a custom to marry those from afar." Among the Bedouin of the Middle East, a young man indeed has the first right to marry his cousin, according to the traditional custom known as *awlād a'mm* (patrilateral parallel marriage). This appears to be a general norm in the Middle East and North Africa (Kressel, 1980). As we already saw, marriage with a relative is also preferred since it is considered to be favorable for the woman's status, with better relationships between the bride and her in-laws. As the young generation emphasizes, this norm has no religious bearing but rather reflects economic and social considerations.

In the following scene, Ismā'īl meets Āysha at the hospital, as if by coincidence. When he tries to open up a conversation, Āysha tells him: "God bless you, Ismā'īl, you know you can't talk to me." Ismā'īl replies: "you know I want you. I came here just to talk to you. It's hard to talk to you in the camp." When Ismā'īl asks his father to approach Āysha's father for the purpose of marriage, his father refuses, saying "we haven't taken brides from them or given them brides in 60 years." But Ismā'īl's father changes his mind following his son's pressure. He organizes a delegation of elders to Āysha's father, who refuses the proposal by saying: "Āysha's cousin [Sāmir] wants her, and if her cousin wants her, I cannot give her to a stranger." His change of heart is brought about by the death of Jamīla's son, and he declares to the men in the *shiqq*: "Cousin marriage causes the birth of deformed, retarded and crazy children. The prophet said we should marry those who are distant."

The caption "End" is followed by the narration: "after Āysha graduated she married Ismā'īl and had four healthy children. Mahmūd married a cousin, and had a sick child. Jamīla, thanks to genetic tests, managed to have a healthy son whom she raised with joy."

The postponing of marriage until after graduation from high school is noteworthy. Educational opportunities for girls are presently impacting two important social realms, age of marriage rates and fertility rates. A rising average age of marriage has important implications for the future of the Bedouin family, as women increasingly see their roles as more diverse than the limited realm of reproduction. While delayed marriage may be viewed by social planners as a positive developmental sign, the older Bedouin generation is concerned by this turn of events.

The 12 script versions of the film embody several important changes that can be grouped under two major categories: the inter-generational conflict and the issue of abortion. A major issue of debate was how to accurately represent the inter-generational conflict while at the same time downplaying it so as not to portray the elders as obsolete. For example, in early script versions Āysha's mother and father were depicted as unanimous in forbidding her marriage to a "stranger." In the final version, the mother (together with her son) is portrayed as negotiating the possibility of an exogamous marriage, while the father objects.

Another issue debated was abortion. Several of the steering committee members argued that abortion should not be mentioned so as not to antagonize religious members of the community. Others, in contrast, said: "selective abortion is the only solution to the problem if the custom of consanguinity persists. If we do not talk about this option then we have nothing to talk about at all" (notes from a steering committee meeting). The compromise, which is reflected in the final script, was to avoid any directive recommendation of abortion. Abortion is implicitly (yet very clearly) mentioned by the doctor. In addition, the script implies a selective abortion made by Jamīla when genetic tests showed that her fetus was affected.

The issues of intergenerational conflict and abortion capture the moral dilemma of nondirectiveness as felt by the health professionals. On the one hand, members argued that their vocation was to reduce the prevalence of hereditary diseases among the Bedouin, and that the film should serve this cause in the most efficient manner. On the other hand, this goal had to be achieved with maximum cultural sensitivity. The moral issue of taking sides and interfering with existing norms, which boils down to the dilemma of nondirectiveness, underpinned the discussions. Premarital carrier matching for "healthy consanguinity," as reflected by the test taken by Āysha and her cousin Mahmūd, represents the essence of the genetic counseling scheme offered to the Bedouin by the local medical center. The romantic, exogamous marriage of Āysha and Ismā'īl represents the wishful thinking of health professionals. In this manner the film catered to the counselors' utilitarian goals that appeared interactionally realizable.

Audience Reception

Based on group discussions conducted at schools with Bedouin pupils and teachers, who saw the film, and the analysis of questionnaires administered to them, premarital carrier matching was found to be positively regarded by the majority of respondents. As I described in the previous chapter, teachers were more positive about genetic counseling (7.65 average on an attitude scale of 1–9). Male and female schoolchildren were also positive, although to a slightly less degree (6.65 and 7, respectively). Below are some excerpts from the transcribed and translated semi-structured group discussions. Four main topics were covered: Authenticity (whether the film was regarded as 'real,' i.e., containing an accurate depiction of reality), consanguinity (pros and cons), genetic tests, and abortion. Below are representative excerpts relating to these themes.

Teachers' and Pupils' Views on the Authenticity and Efficiency of the Film

Teachers and pupils agreed, in principle, that the problems depicted in the film were real. They also agreed that the solutions offered in the film (i.e., genetic tests, exogamous marriage, and selective abortion) were not commonly practiced by the Bedouin. In a sense, the real question was not if the film was perceived as 'authentic' but whether it was effective. It was obvious to the filmmakers and the health professionals that their script did not mean to be authentic but rather to stage an 'authentic' drama that relays the required message. However, the question of authenticity was also relevant to efficiency. If the script were perceived as too fictive or far-fetched, this would no doubt limit its effectiveness.

> Everyone knows there are a lot of familial diseases in the community. But it is very rare to do a test for such diseases. [Teacher]

The film is interesting but it cannot change what we do, because what we do depends on our parents. [Pupil]
This film is for uneducated Bedouin who live in tents in the desert, not for city Bedouin. [Pupil]
A Bedouin girl will not marry to a stranger or to someone who comes from a distant place. How can this thing happen? Our girls are at home or at school. They cannot meet strangers. This rarely happens. [Teacher]
The pain and suffering that are supposed to affect a child with genetic disease are not emphasized in the film. Jamīla's sick son looks quite normal. We are not told the name of his sickness. [Teacher]
Jamīla's son is not a good example of a painful genetic disease. We are just told that he has a disease, and then we are told that he died because of it. [Pupil]
They should have shown the daily suffering of a family with a child that has genetic diseases, otherwise it is not convincing. [Pupil]
The change of heart of the elders is unexpected. Āysha's father and Ismā'īl's father both change their mind and let the youngsters do as they please. This would not happen in real life. [Teacher]
My father controls the family. Especially the daughters in it. I wouldn't dream of acting like Āysha. [Pupil]
When Āysha's father changes his mind following the death of Jamīla's son, it is too sudden. He sits with the men in the tent and declares: I accept Ismā'īl's and Ayasha's marriage. Everyone else objects, including the youngsters of the family, who are supposed to belong to the generation that wants to make a difference in the old customs. [Teacher]
Do we want to take care of genetic tests or of family affairs? The film mixes these two problems. There is the problem of tests and the problem of marriage between clans. This is too much in one film. It was too much drama, and too little instruction [Teacher]
It is not wise to show how Āysha and Ismā'īl meet "as if by coincidence" at the hospital. This is against the norms. When a man wants to marry someone, he must not speak to her directly. [Teacher]
You are presenting the hospital as a place where unmarried men and women can meet and speak. Elders who see this will forbid their daughters to go to the hospital without inspection. [Teacher]
You are putting a stigma on the hospital as a place of secret meeting for lovers. [Teacher]

Perceptions of Consanguinity

As the group was urged by the moderator to reflect about the pros and cons of consanguinity, the following themes emerged among both teachers and pupils:

Pros

- Keeping family ties, keeping the family together. Many cited in this context the Bedouin proverb "helping your cousin get off her horse" which means that young men have the first right to marry their cousin.
- It is difficult/impossible to find a groom outside the family.
- Cousin marriage helps keep the family property inside the family. When you give out a daughter of the family, you also give out family property.
- Consanguinity helps to keep the woman's honor. Even if the man hates his wife, he will not hit her if she's his cousin. He will not shame her.
- Cousin marriage provides a practical solution for "old maids" that have a marriage problem.

Cons

- Cousin marriage is bad because of all these genetic defects and diseases.
- To marry those who are distant is good. This is the word of the prophet. It also brings together distant families and makes them closer.
- In these days it is much more common to marry out of love, romantic marriages, and not pre-arranged marriage.

Attitudes of pupils could be further subsumed under three categories: modern, traditional, and hybrid. The modern category, comprised almost entirely of boys, included those who were opposed to cousin marriage as a form of family paternalism. A typical "modern" attitude stated that "in our times, our families can no longer decide for us whom we are going to marry. I will make this decision for myself, whether it is a cousin or a distant person" (spoken by a boy). While aware of the "genetic risk" in consanguinity, this attitude also emphasized the quest for individualism and romantic love. This category represented a minority of the pupils (about 20%). Notwithstanding its possible naïveté, the existence of this attitude could be an indication of social change among the Bedouin.

Second, the traditional category, with more girls than boys, stressed the normative importance of cousin marriage through the above-mentioned repertoire of "pros." While these pupils said they understood the genetic risk of consanguinity, they also stressed its functional aspects in terms of culture, economy, and the family interest. This category represented the majority of pupils (about 60%).

Third, the hybrid category, held by boys and girls, sought a reconciliation of genetic counseling and traditional norms. A typical compromise-seeking attitude stated that "it is difficult and anti-tradition to marry girls outside the family, but it is also important to do the test before deciding on cousin marriage." Or: "it is not in contradiction, cousin marriage and genetic testing. It is not bad to marry your cousin, but you should do the test first." This attitude matched the program's rationale of "healthy consanguinity," namely cousin marriage based on carrier matching.

The teachers, many of them Arabs from the northern part of Israel rather than local Bedouin, were mostly in favor of the first, modern category. This was in line with their role as agents of socialization but also reflected the external viewpoint they had on the local Bedouin population. Many of them assumed a critical and paternalist tone. As one of the teachers said: "even if we believe that cousin marriage is a norm from the past, the locals are not going to give up on it so quickly. It is going to take a generation [i.e., about 20 years] before there is a noticeable change."

Genetic Tests

For many of the pupils, the depiction of carrier matching in the film was not clear enough. Because the actual procedure of blood drawing and genetic testing was not shown, and the emphasis was on "taking the test together," this gave some of the pupils a wrong impression about the actual procedure. Other students expressed anxiety about the negative implications of genetic tests, both in terms of their parents' objection and in terms of potential stigmatization. While expressing a positive view regarding genetic testing, especially in the context of carrier matching and "healthy consanguinity," the teachers were pessimistic about the actual uptake of genetic testing by the Bedouin due to the negative image and potentially negative consequences of the tests.

> It is very difficult to persuade couples to do a genetic test. Even if you and I agree that a test can be good. In reality, it is seen as something that causes problems. [Teacher]
>
> The film presents a situation in which the tests have very difficult consequences for those who take it. Āysha could not marry her cousin Mahmūd, because they were found to be carriers in the test. This is a negative consequence. Why not show us a positive consequence

> where two cousins are found to be compatible and get married after taking the test? [Teacher]
> We are told that Āysha and Mahmūd took the test together. Does it mean that they were examined together? I mean, a simultaneous physical test? This is very difficult to believe. I can hardly believe that a girl would accept being physically examined in front of her fiancé. [Pupil]
> It was not clear from the film what kind of test they took. [Pupil]
> Genetic tests appear to be a good idea if there are specific tests for the disease that is in your family. The film was not specific enough about this.[Teacher]
> Our parents tell us that all diseases are from God. It is in God's power to kill a man at every moment.[Pupil]
> I am too young to decide for myself. My parents do not understand these biological concepts that we study at school, so if I tell them, they'll say it's all in God's hands.[Pupil]
> If people hear you did a genetic test they will start asking questions. They will become suspicious and say you are sick yourself. [Pupil]
> Genetic tests are the only solution for the problem because the norm of cousin marriage is too strong. Consanguinity will not go away. You cannot tell us to go marry other people. What you can do is use these tests to tell us who is compatible and who is not. If this person's genes do not match his cousin's, then they shouldn't marry. Take their chance with another cousin. This way you'll reduce the risk of having sick children. [Teacher]

Abortion

Both the pupils and the teachers found the issue of abortion to be sensitive and many of them worried that it should not be discussed at school. Although the teachers acknowledged the importance of the issue and some thought that pupils should be taught about the variety of views within Muslim religion about abortion, still they were hesitant about bringing up the issue in class. The majority of pupils responded that abortion was not a viable option due to religion and custom.

> There are several Muslim views on the matter of abortion, some are more liberal and some are stringent. People are not aware of this. They don't know what to do in case of an affected fetus. They will go and ask their local *Qadi* (religious guide). Some *Qadi* will tell you that

abortion is forbidden unless the mother's health is at stake. But I also heard about a *fatwa* [religious instruction] that it is okay to abort in the first four months of pregnancy. [Teacher]

School is not the right place to talk about tests that lead to abortion. If my father heard that we talk about this at school, he would forbid me to go to school. [Pupil]

If I was pregnant and the doctors told me I had a defected baby, I would not abort. This is against religion. [Pupil]

If I was married to a cousin and we had genetic diseases in the family, I would do tests during pregnancy. I would do the early test, and I would do it secretly, in a distant hospital, so that nobody in the family knows about it. [Pupil]

It is better not to speak about abortion openly. I cannot simply raise the issue with my parents, they will think something is wrong with me. [Pupil]

To Match or Not To Match?

Interviews with teachers and pupils were instructive in terms of how the film could be improved. Respondents made useful remarks concerning the authenticity and efficiency of the film, the balance between drama and instruction, the need to portray more vividly the painful experience of living with genetic disease, and the inadvertent stigmatization of the hospital as a meeting place for young lovers. These remarks illustrate the benefit of conducting focus groups with the target audience, preferably in a stage when the script is still under work.

The film illustrates two major points of collision between the traditional culture of the Bedouin population and the modern, biomedical culture of health services. Both of these issues, the intergenerational conflict and abortion, capture the moral dilemma of nondirectiveness as felt by the health professionals involved. Within the community, there was no consensus on these issues. First, there was no Muslim consensus regarding the permissibility of abortion. Second, the inter-generational conflict was an existing social reality in a population that since the 1950s and increasingly after 1967 has been undergoing a rapid process of transition from a semi-nomadic to a sedentary, westernized way of life and was lacking a centralized authority structure.

The attitudes of respondents presented a dichotomous picture in regard to these two contested issues. On the one hand, there were pupils whose comments reflected their dependence on family and tradition. On the other hand most of the teachers as well as many pupils regarded the film's message positively and suggested ways to improve its efficiency. The data indicate that respondents understood that consanguinity could lead to the birth of impaired children. Interestingly, respondents did not argue that both the consequences of consanguinity and the tests are uncertain in their outcomes—a claim that was found, for example, in a study of Bedouin women's selective use of prenatal screening (Lewando-Hundt et al., 2001).

An overly critical reading of the film 'Āysha' would focus on its directiveness as eugenic. The film's documentary pretense could also be targeted as the epitome of an "imagined genetic community." The allusion is to Benedict Anderson's (1983) "imagined community," which stands for the power of collective representations to make possible imagined communities made up of people whom one could assume were "just like us." Popular notions of genetics are quite pertinent to ethnicity and nationhood, since "genes" are imagined as representing one's biological (ethnic, racial) essence (Simpson, 2000). In a similar manner, the documentary presentation of 'Āysha' could be critically read as a narrative for a new Bedouin community, imagined by health professionals, where actors replace community members and staged authenticity replaces social reality. However, the analysis of audience reception shows that community members, while being critical towards rather than captivated by the film, still identified with its basic message to a large extent.

'Āysha' can also be read as reflecting and promoting a change in the traditional role of Bedouin women. Āysha, the heroine, personifies a new role model for young Bedouin women. She disobeys her father, refuses to be given to her cousins, and finally marries a stranger after her high school graduation. In Bedouin terms, Āysha is a feminist rebel. While the lives of many Bedouin men are increasingly impacted by external interactions, the division of realms (domestic sphere/external sphere) based upon gender and age persists, and seclusion and social restrictions on women remain largely in place (Dinero, 1997). The state of concealment of women (*haram*) to ensure marriage with other agnates is particularly strong in Bedouin society (Mernissi, 1987).

Negev Bedouin women currently experience a time of transformation. In resettled urban settings, they are increasingly forced into a more domestic home mode with full child-care responsibilities; at the same time, they are cut off from the numerous responsibilities that they held in the nomadic arena. Women's closer proximity to non-agnatic males (that is, males who are not close relatives) is perceived as a growing threat to tradition. This was indicated by the widely shared rejection, among respondents, of using the hospital as a rendezvous point for Āysha and Ismā'īl. The film can thus be read as an attempt to empower Bedouin women.

Nondirectiveness and Its Lay Interpretations

The film's positive reception by Bedouin respondents sheds new light on the professional dilemma of nondirectiveness. Discussions in focus groups have shown that respondents interpreted the film's message as directive, irrespective of its intended meaning. Moreover, this interpretation was normative for Bedouin respondents. The Bedouin respondents' bias for directiveness was also apparent in their common attitude regarding the ineffective portrayal of the genetic disease in the film. Many of the respondents (teachers as well as pupils) stressed that in order to be effective and have an impact, the film should have presented the pains and difficulties of living with a genetic disease much more vividly. Many respondents suggested that when discussing the film at school, pictures of people affected by severe genetic diseases should be shown and explained. It appears that while the educational rationale behind the film sought to (or at least was sensitive to) avoid intimidation and directiveness, this was what the local audience expected and looked for. However, such hypothesis regarding the community's expectation for directiveness required further empirical testing.

To evaluate the effects of ethnicity, culture and counseling style on the interpretation of nondirectiveness in genetic counseling, a questionnaire containing premarital and prenatal case vignettes in two versions (pessimistic/optimistic) was administered to 281 Jewish and 133 Bedouin respondents. The first study population was comprised of Jewish students enrolled in a university and a community college in the Negev (southern part of Israel). The second study population was comprised of Muslim-Bedouin college students from the same area.

The purpose of this study was to evaluate the interpretation of optimistic versus pessimistic genetic counseling vignettes in two distinct cultural groups, and to determine if there were differences between these two groups in the interpretation of what was being said. In targeting these two groups, I expected the interpretation of Jewish students to be more consistent with the espoused message (i.e., nondirectiveness) of counselors. Bedouin students, in contrast, were expected to interpret the message as directive, due to traditional norms. In addition, I distinguished between two groups of Jewish students: university and community college. This was done in order to explore whether culture (Jewish vs. Bedouin) or education (University vs. Community College) were key factors in differences in response. If the difference in interpretation between Jewish and Bedouin students would overshadow the difference between University and college students (within the Jewish group), this could be more confidentially attributed to cultural-religious factors, rather than academic background.

Questionnaire Development

A 23-item questionnaire that included two scenarios (case vignettes) of premarital and prenatal genetic counseling was developed. Each scenario presented a concrete dilemma (see Appendix) while quoting a counselor as the source of information. Respondents were asked after each scenario how they interpret the counselor's words and what they would do in such a situation. Following the two scenarios, the questionnaire concluded with a general query regarding the primary goal of genetic counseling. The counselor's words that appeared in the questionnaire were chosen based on interviews with counselors at the local medical center. A pilot study involving six genetic counselors took place to confirm the validity of the questionnaire. The scenarios were modified until all counselors agreed that the scenarios correctly represented their manner of speech in similar situations. It was found that while all counselors agreed on the basic format and sequence of information, there was variability in terms of tone. Some chose a more optimistic tone while others were more pessimistic. For example, some preferred a more optimistic assertion such as "the test shows you still have 75 percent chance in each pregnancy to give birth to a healthy child," while others chose the more pessimistic phrase "the test shows you have 25 percent risk in each pregnancy to give birth to an affected child." To examine the effect of optimism/pessimism, two versions (one using optimistic phrases and the other pessimistic) were constructed and randomly administered to respondents. The resulting questions were in a multiple-choice format. When presented with the final two versions, all counselors' selections were identical, confirming the reliability of the questionnaire.

The Use of Optimistic vs. Pessimistic Questionnaire Versions

The use of optimistic vs. pessimistic questionnaire versions was not part of the original research design. Rather, it was added as a result of the pilot stage in which, during questionnaire development, it was found that some counselors used optimistic assertions while other used pessimistic ones. The two questionnaire versions were constructed in order to explore the effect of counseling style on interpretation. I expected the pessimistic version to correlate with more directive interpretations as compared to the optimistic version, across all groups. For example, people who hear a negative description of the fetus' condition are likely to interpret this as a recommendation to abort. Optimism, in itself, can also be construed as directive, most likely in a positive way. In the options provided to respondents, however, the only "positive" choice was the item that represented the nondirective message of genetic counseling. In that sense, the optimistic version was thought to be construed as "less directive" and to coincide with a higher level of interpretation of the intended message, as compared to the pessimistic version.

Study Recruitment and Questionnaire Administration

Questionnaires were presented, in Hebrew and Arabic, to 145 Jewish university students (JUS), 136 Jewish community college students (JCC), and 133 Bedouin community college students (BCC). All questionnaires were anonymous. They did, however, include basic socio-demographic data regarding sex, age, susceptibility (having a relative who is affected by a genetic disease), religious denomination (Jewish, Muslim or other) and religiosity (orthodox, traditional and secular). Respondents represented a random sample of undergraduate students in the humanities and social sciences, and had not been previously selected for counseling or genetics education. The JUS group was recruited from the local University (Ben-Gurion University of the Negev), while the JCC and BCC groups were recruited from two local community colleges. Selection for the academic program in which JUS were enrolled was competitive and based on previous academic achievements (high psychometric and matriculation grades), and many in the JUS group came from the urban center of Israel. The JCC group was mostly from the local periphery of the Negev, had poorer academic background in terms of psychometric and matriculation grades (an average 200 points less in the standard academic psychometric test, as compared to JUS), and a slightly lower socio-economic status. The BCC group was from the Negev, had a slightly poorer academic background as compared to JCC and a lower socio-economic status. All students were recruited from large introductory courses and the different versions (pessimistic/optimistic) were randomly administered. There was no incentive for participation. Having received the agreement of the lecturer, the research assistants administered the questionnaires about 10 minutes before the end of class. An explanation regarding the purpose of the study was given by one of the research assistants, stressing that questionnaires are anonymous and do not relate in any way to the coursework. Questionnaire results were analyzed using SPSS statistics software (SPSS 11.0 for Windows, 15 Nov. 2001, (c) SPSS, Inc.). Comparisons of questionnaire scores among groups were performed using chi-square analysis and a difference of $p<0.05$ was considered significant.

Table 7. Socio-Demographic Characteristics of the Study Sample

Group	JUS	JCC	BCC
N	145	136	133
Religion	Jewish	Jewish	Muslim
Religiosity	95% secular 5% traditional	93% secular 7% traditional	3% secular 44% traditional 53% orthodox
Susceptibility (having an affected relative)	9%	17%	23%
Gender	66% F, 44% M	69% F, 31% M	76% F, 24% M
Age (mean)	23.12	22.4	20.3

Results

Responses to the questions were interpreted in the following manner. All the questions contained one item that represented the espoused nondirective message of genetic counseling. These items, which were validated by the genetic counselors who participated in the pilot stage, are italicized in all the ensuing tables. The nondirective items were: (1) "In case you get married, it is recommended that you test the fetus in each pregnancy in order to have all the information and make your own decision"; (2) "the only message is to consider all the information and reach my own informed decision"; and (3) The primary goal of genetic counseling is "providing information to counselees so that they can reach their own informed decision".

During 2002 the questionnaire was administered in the three pre-selected settings. Groups were quite homogenous in terms of religious denomination and practice (which are often different in Israel since many are born Jewish and keep this denomination yet in practice consider themselves to be secular). Table 7 presents the demographics of the study sample.

The Effect of Ethnicity and Culture. Selection of the nondirective item in all questions was much higher in JUS and JCC in relation to BCC (see figures 1 and 2). This pattern was consistent across all three questions as well as the two questionnaire versions. The differences between Jewish and Bedouin students' selections were significant across all questions. This pattern validates the hypothesis regarding the effect of ethnicity and culture on the interpretation of nondirectiveness. Gender and susceptibility did not present a significant or predictable effect on selections within groups.

The differences within the Jewish group, which were always smaller than the difference between the Jewish and Bedouin groups, did not present a predictable pattern. In the first (premarital) scenario, more JUS than JCC selected

Figure 5. Interpretation of Nondirectiveness Measured by Percent of Selections in Each Group, Version 1 ("Pessimistic")

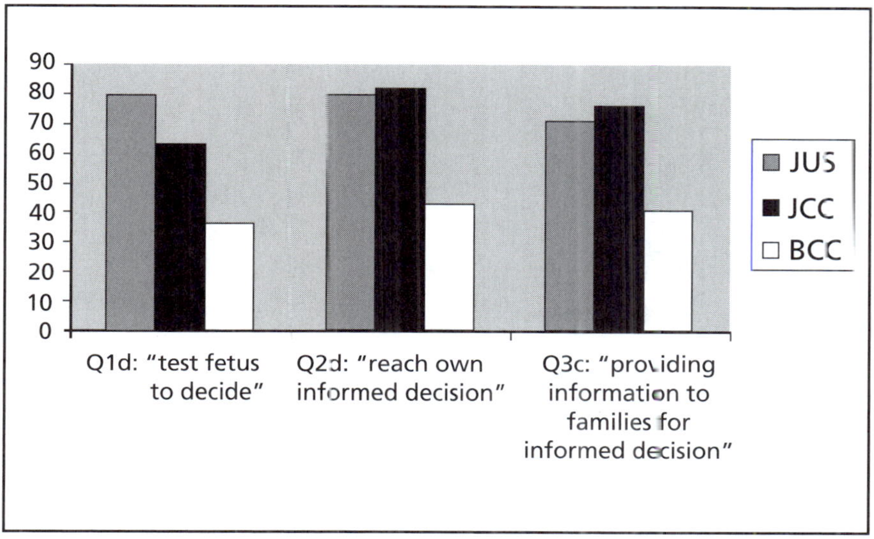

Figure 6. Interpretation of Nondirectiveness Measured by Percent of Selections in Each Group, Version 2 ("Optimistic")

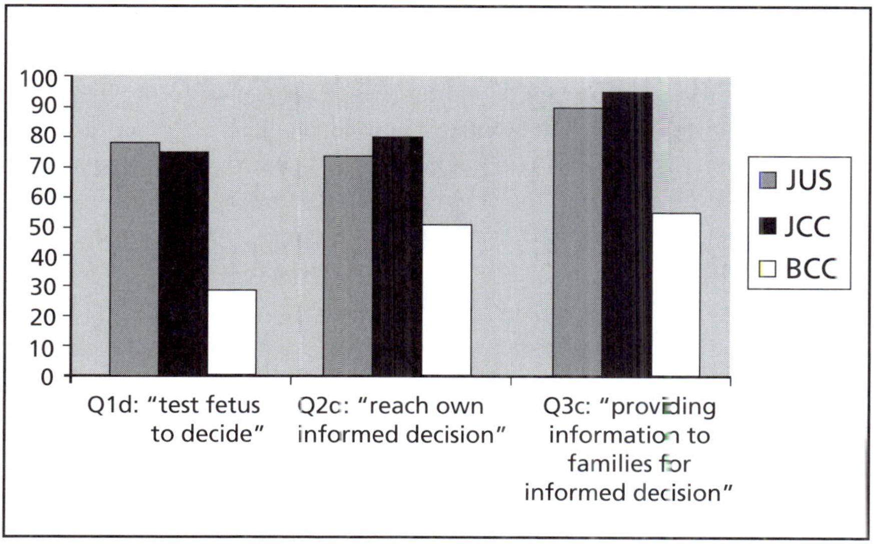

the nondirective items. In the second (prenatal) scenario, a smaller number of JUS, as compared to JCC, selected the nondirective items. While the percent of abortion-seeking BCC respondents is still low in comparison to JUS and JCC, it nevertheless presents a marked potential for social change in the traditional Bedouin community, where there is a widely-accepted Muslim ban on abortion. In the first (premarital) scenario, the option of abortion was significantly downplayed (see tables 8 and 9). This is due to the option of partner switching, which was selected by a majority of in BCC.

A majority of Jewish respondents preferred to "marry current partner and test the fetus in each pregnancy." In contrast, a majority of Bedouin respondents preferred to switch partners as a result of the genetic test. This represents a more directive interpretation and a preventive intention to switch partners. Jewish students rarely selected these items. The different match between interpretation and intention—nondirective and open-ended versus directive and preventive in the case of Jewish and Bedouin, respectively—once again highlights the effect of cultural norms.

The Effect of Counseling Style. In comparing the pessimistic and optimistic versions of the questionnaire, counseling style was not found to have a statistically significant effect on interpretation, within as well as across the study groups (see tables 8 and 9). Analysis of the general (third) question, regarding the primary goal of genetic counseling, showed that the majority in all study groups interpreted the role of counseling as nondirective. There was a statistically significant difference in the selection patterns between Jewish and Bedouin respondents. In addition, there was a statistically significant difference between the pessimistic and optimistic versions across study groups (see table 10). The distribution of selections in this question supports the view that nondirectiveness is contingent on cultural norms as well as counseling style.

Nondirectiveness has been discussed from ideological and practical angles that focus on the message of genetic counseling. The survey reported here focused, in contrast, on the complementary aspect of interpretation. The findings show that when provided to university and college Jewish students, whose norms are modern and Western-like, the nondirective message of counseling was interpreted as intended by the majority. Some have suggested that nondirectiveness, as a Western ideal, is both irrelevant and unattainable in non-Western contexts. This suggestion finds support in the finding that Bedouin students, representing a traditional and religious ethnic minority in Israel, interpreted counseling in a more directive manner.

This study also examined the effect of counseling style on interpretation. I hypothesized the pessimistic version to correlate with more directive interpretations as compared to the optimistic version, across all groups. This

Table 8. Selections of Jewish and Bedouin Students in the "Pessimistic" Version

BCC N=61	JCC N=68	JUS N=66	
			How do you interpret the counselor's words (premarital scenario):
21(34%)	6(9%)	3(5%)	Seek out another partner who does not carry the mutation
1(2)%	3(4%)	3(5%)	In case you get married, adopt children
9(15%)	16(24%)	8(12%)	In case you get married, you'll have to test the fetus in each pregnancy, and abort in case s/he is affected
22(36%)	*43(63%)*	*52(79%)*	*In case you get married, it is recommended that you test the fetus in each pregnancy in order to have all the information and make your own decision*
8(13%)	0	0	You can get married and forget the whole thing

Difference Statistic:

JUS–JCC	χ^2=4.46	e=0.03	power < .2
Jewish-Bedouin	χ^2=48.16**	e=0.24	power > .99

BCC N=61	JCC N=68	JUS N=66	
			If it were up to you, what do you intend to do in this situation:
29(48%)	7(10%)	2(3%)	Seek a partner who does not carry the gene for Tay-Sachs
	4(6%)	6(9%)	Marry current partner and adopt children
8(13%)	22(32%)	30(46%)	Marry current partner while being aware that if the fetus is affected, you'll have an abortion
20(33%)	35(51%)	28(42%)	Marry current partner and test the fetus in each pregnancy
4(7%)	0	0	Marry current partner and forget the whole thing

Difference Statistic:

JUS–JCC	χ^2=5.1	e=0.03	power < .2
Jewish-Bedouin	χ^2=60.24**	e=0.3	power > .99

BCC N=61	JCC N=68	JUS N=66	
			How do you interpret the counselor's words (prenatal scenario):
21(34%)	6(9%)	3(5%)	A recommendation to terminate the pregnancy
7(11%)	5(7%)	10(15%)	No clear recommendation, but the counselor would prefer that I choose to abort
7(11%)	1(2%)	0	No clear recommendation, but the counselor would prefer that I continue with the pregnancy
26(43%)	*56(82%)*	*53(80%)*	*The only message is to consider all the information and reach my own informed decision*

Table 8 (*continued*)

Difference Statistic:

JUS–JCC	χ^2=3.72	e=0.02	power < .1
Jewish-Bedouin	χ^2=41.96**	e=0.21	power > .99

			If it were up to you, what do you intend to do in this situation:
22(36%)	31(46%)	40(61%)	Terminate the pregnancy
13(21%)	4(6%)	4(6%)	Continue with the pregnancy
26(43%)	33(48%)	22(33%)	I don't know

Difference Statistic:

JUS–JCC	χ^2=3.28	e=0.02	power < .1
Jewish-Bedouin	χ^2=11.73**	e=0.06	power = 0.6

* $p < 0.05$ (percents are rounded)
** $p < 0.005$
Power analysis for the χ^2 test was computed using **e**, the effect size index (Cohen, 1969: 242–50)

hypothesis was refuted in the context of the two scenarios. However, counseling style had a significant impact on interpretation in the general (third) question regarding the primary goal of genetic counseling. In this question, the majority of respondents in all groups selected the nondirective item (Q3c—The primary goal of genetic counseling is "providing information to counselees so that they can reach their own informed decision"). The pessimistic version significantly lowered the percentage of this item in all groups. I therefore suggest that pessimistic counseling tends to compromise the counselee's sense of nondirectiveness. This finding is important in implying that how the counselor speaks does make a difference (see also Pilnick, 2002; Chapple and May, 1996; Chapple, Campion & May, 1997; Dunne and Warren, 1998). Counselors should therefore avoid a pessimistic tone if they wish to be interpreted as nondirective. However, findings are not consistent in this matter, as the two scenarios did not present a similar effect.

The Bedouin as an Interpretive Community

Some have suggested that nondirectiveness, as a Western ideal, is both irrelevant and unattainable in non-Western contexts. Mittman et al. (1998: 62–63) report how Asian-Pacific and Latin American immigrants who participated in

Table 9. Selections of Jewish and Bedouin Students in the "Optimistic" Version

BCC N=72	JCC N=68	JUS N=79	
			How do you interpret the counselor's words (premarital scenario):
33(46%)	1(1%)	2(3%)	Seek out another partner who does not carry the mutation
5(7)%	0	1(1%)	In case you get married, adopt children
10(14%)	16(24%)	14(18%)	In case you get married, you'll have to test the fetus in each pregnancy, and abort in case s/he is affected
20*(28%)*	*51(75%)*	*62(78%)*	*In case you get married, it is recommended that you test the fetus in each pregnancy in order to have all the information and make your own decision*
4(6%)	0	0	You can get married and forget the whole thing

Difference Statistic:

JUS–JCC	χ^2=1.71	e=0.01	power < 1
Pessimistic–Optimistic (total)	χ^2=1.35**	e=0.003	power > 1
Jewish-Bedouin	χ^2=113.94**	e=0.52	power > .99

			If it were up to you, what do you intend to do in this situation:
22(31%)	2(3%)	2(3%)	Seek a partner who does not carry the gene for Tay-Sachs
4(5%)	2(3%)	3(4%)	Marry current partner and adopt children
15(21%)	28(41%)	49(62%)	Marry current partner while being aware that if the fetus is affected, you'll have an abortion
25(35%)	35(52%)	24(30%)	Marry current partner and test the fetus in each pregnancy
6(8%)	1(1%)	1(1%)	Marry current partner and forget the whole thing

Difference Statistic:

JUS–JCC	χ^2=7.13	e=0.04	power < .1
Jewish-Bedouin	χ^2=50.16**	e=0.22	power > .99

			How do you interpret the counselor's words (prenatal scenario):
17(24%)	5(7%)	3(4%)	A recommendation to terminate the pregnancy
15(21%)	7(10%)	18(23%)	No clear recommendation, but the counselor would prefer that I choose to abort
4(5%)	1(1%)	1(1%)	No clear recommendation, but the counselor would prefer that I continue with the pregnancy
36*(50%)*	*55(81%)*	*57(72%)*	*The only message is to consider all the information and reach my own informed decision*

Table 9 (*continued*)

Difference Statistic:

JUS–JCC	χ^2=4.56	e=0.03	power < .2
Pessimistic–Optimistic (total)	χ^2=5.16**	e=0.01	power > .6
Jewish-Bedouin	χ^2=21.21**	e=0.09	power = .91

			If it were up to you, what do you intend to do in this situation:
32(44%)	31(46%)	47(59%)	Terminate the pregnancy
14(19%)	9(13%)	6(8%)	Continue with the pregnancy
26(36%)	28(41%)	26(33%)	I don't know

Difference Statistic:

JUS–JCC	χ^2=3.13	e=0.02	power < .1
Jewish-Bedouin	χ^2=3.8**	e=0.01	power < .1

* $p < 0.05$
** $p < 0.005$

Table 10. Selections of Jewish and Bedouin Students Regarding the Goal of Counseling

Cross Tabulated by counseling style (P= pessimistic, O= optimistic)

BCC		JCC		JUS		
O	P	O	P	O	P	
18(25%)	18(29%)	3(4%)	9(13%)	6(8%)	10(15%)	Avoiding the birth of an affected baby
12(17%)	18(29%)	2(3%)	7(10%)	3(4%)	9(14%)	Reducing the number of deleterious genes in the population
42(58%)	25(41%)	63(93%)	52(76%)	70(89%)	47(71%)	Providing information to families so they can reach an informed decision.

Difference Statistic:

JUS–JCC	(Pessimistic Version)	χ^2=0.73	e=0.005	power <.1
	(Optimistic Version)	χ^2=1.23	e=0.008	power <.1
Jewish-Bedouin	(Pessimistic Version)	χ^2=29.14**	e=0.13	power = .95
	(Optimistic Version)	χ^2=33.18**	e=0.17	power = .99

Pessimistic-Optimistic (JUS)	χ^2= 7.38*	e = 0.05	.25< power < .5
Pessimistic-Optimistic (JCC)	χ^2= 6.8*	e = 0.05	.25< power < .5
Pessimistic-Optimistic (BCC)	χ^2= 4.59*	e = 0.03	.25< power < .5
Pessimistic-Optimistic (total)	χ^2= 14.56**	e = 0.03	power = .95

cross-cultural genetics education and used amniocentesis in San Francisco often asked for the counselors' opinion and seemed to be at a loss when a clear direction was not provided. Moreover, about 35% of the study participants were unaware of the voluntary nature of amniocentesis. The authors recount how "ironically, adhering to our nondirective counseling left our clients searching for answers from individuals less knowledgeable than us; their parents in-law, their immigration sponsors, or neighborhood herbalist" (ibid., p. 62).

Sociolinguistic and anthropological studies have shown how interpretation can depend on group characteristics and norms (Fish, 1980). The question of what caused the differences in interpretation between Jewish-Israeli and Arab-Bedouin respondents is open for conjectures. I argue that it was a different underlying worldview or cultural narrative (Britton and Pellegrini, 1991). Generally speaking, the relevant interpretive norms of Jewish-Israelis—especially the young Jewish-Israeli generation—stem from a cultural narrative built on Western-like secularism, self-reliance and individualism (Katriel, 1986; Hazan, 2000). Such a worldview generates an expectation for nondirectiveness. In contrast, the relevant interpretive norms of the Bedouin—including the younger generation—represent a cultural narrative underpinned by collectivism, tradition, and patriarchy (Mernissi, 1987). The Bedouin worldview therefore reflects an expectation for directiveness. The Bedouin community is underpinned by kinship ties, patriarchy and religion to an extent no longer characteristic of modern Western societies. Values such as authority, obligation, honor and caring are all family-centered rather than individual. Such a worldview generates an expectation for directiveness. Bedouin socialization focuses on social sanctions and conformity rather than individual decision-making in the context of family planning (see Kressel, 1986, 1992). In addition, Bedouin religious norms such as the ban on abortion largely preclude an individual choice of prenatal genetic test.

The cultural context of interpretation highlights the need to embed analyses of genetic counseling within local communities rather than merely concentrating on two-person interactions. The individual level, which concerns the patient-counselor interaction, often depends on community-level norms such as patriarchy, consanguinity, or religious banning of abortion, which characterize the Bedouin. The Bedouin interpretation of the counselor's words as a recommendation to seek out a partner who is not a carrier of the mutation is clearly related to the existence of a religious ban on abortion. Furthermore, the Bedouin encounter with the Israeli medical establishment is commonly framed by authoritative and paternalistic relations (Lewando-Hundt et al., 2001). The Bedouin interpretation of the counselor's words as directive can be seen as a corollary of this experience.

In the first (premarital) scenario, the majority of Bedouin students selected the option of partner switching due to genetic risk. Jewish-Israeli students, in contrast, rejected this option. This finding implies that carrier-screening programs implemented in traditional ethnic communities, likely to be perceived as coercive by Western standards, may be culturally adapted to the norms and preferences of community members. Programs like *Dor Yeshorim*, whose success is documented, are also quite directive. For Western observers, they highlight the ethical problem of free choice in a directive environment and of claiming that individuals are "autonomous" whereas their framework for decision-making has already been constructed by health professionals (Hoedemaekers and ten Have, 1998). The findings of this study, in contrast, highlight the possible match between these programs' rationale and the norms of community members. Mittman et al. (1998: 67), who were involved in counseling to Latin and Asian-Pacific immigrants in the San Francisco area, conclude that "counselors should attempt to provide genetic information in a manner which recognizes and respects clients' life experiences and cultural conviction." Sometimes this may also involve a modification of the Western ideal of nondirectiveness.

The implications of this study suggest that misinterpretation of meaning based on cultural differences is likely to happen when counseling to traditional ethnic minorities. The message of counseling, for example, is likely to be interpreted by such communities as directive in regard to partner selection, abortion and family planning. While this may be seen as an ethical compromise by a liberal-universalist approach, it is supported by a communitarian view that bioethics are local (Tan Alora and Lumitao, 2001; Hoshino, 1997). Counselors can use similar or modified questionnaires or scenario-based interviews in order to elicit the attitudes and interpretations of specific communities with religious/traditional norms that affect counseling, such as a religious ban on abortion or consanguinity. It is possible that the vignettes used for this study have themselves been influenced by the culture in which they were developed. The material in both scenarios is probably different than what would typically be done in the U.S.A. To study this cultural difference, data is required concerning the reactions of North American genetic counselors to these vignettes, and how they would typically be done in the U.S.A.

The analysis of responses in the context of the film as well as in the context of the questionnaire with the genetic counseling scenarios illustrates a common Bedouin disposition for directiveness. This finding was replicated in these two different studies in which different stimuli and different research methods were employed. It was validated by both qualitative (the focus groups) and quantitative (the questionnaire) analyses. What are we to make of this finding concerning the Bedouin disposition for authority and directiveness? This finding does not mean that the Bedouin prefer to be told what to do by health care professionals, or that the Bedouin will necessarily comply with what they are being told. Indeed, the patterns of utilization observed in this study demonstrate the opposite. The finding concerning the Bedouin disposition for authority and directiveness does suggest, however, that the Bedouin are likely to interpret the messages of health care professionals (genetic counselors included) as directive irrespective of the way these messages are being phrased. Indeed, many of the Bedouin respondents commented in the context of the film that in order to be effective, genetics education should be even more directive, making use of alarming photos and fear-provoking descriptions of the difficult consequences of genetic diseases to the affected individual, their relatives and the community. In considering the practical implications of this finding, the dilemma for health professionals is, therefore, whether to remain loyal to the standard ethical code of non-directiveness (which according to my findings is misinterpreted in any event), or to be intentionally directive for the sake of efficiency, as many of the Bedouin respondents suggested. In the end of the day, one's solution to this dilemma depends on how one solves the inherent conflict between the values of non-directiveness and medical efficiency, and whether one gives priority to local communal norms or to the cosmopolitan view of western bioethics. I continue to discuss this important issue in the following chapter, which provides a conclusion for the book.

Conclusion: Beyond a Western Bioethics? The Future of Community Genetics

Conducted in the interstices of tradition and medicalization, this study was perhaps expected to demonstrate the set of barriers and problems that it did. Several focal points of conflict were highlighted in the ethnography, including difficulties relating to Western bioethical practices such as patient autonomy and informed consent; difficulty grasping the concept of genetic inheritance, genetic diagnosis and genetic risk; cultural beliefs regarding childbearing and match making; family dynamics that are unfamiliar to the genetic counselor and a mismatch between public and private arenas of negotiation. These issues are not unique to the Bedouin community but rather characterize cross-cultural genetic counseling in general (Weil and Mittman, 1993; Sue and Sue, 1990; Wang and Marsh, 1992). Health professionals may be too easily tempted to perceive such "barriers" and "difficulties" as the result of cultural differences and an unbridgeable gap in mentalities. However, a closer ethnographic analysis may prove that many of the difficulties are the result of micro-political circumstances and personal agendas. What appears in Western eyes to be the result of scientific ignorance and "traditional mentality" may prove to be the result of practical wit in the face of community and personal constraints. Indeed, the data show that many Bedouin understood the message of genetics, but used it for their own interests.

The meaning of counseling differed for participants. The counselors and other professionals involved in the program negotiated the compromising of ethical standards through the rhetoric of cultural adaptation. The adaptation to the norms of the community was seen as a pragmatic trade-off whose success should be evaluated. This professional arena of negotiation was not communicated to counselees. Furthermore, professionals did not have identical views on this matter. Even among Bedouin health professionals there were competing perspectives on how best to represent and empower the community. Bedouin counselees, on their part, also had private agendas that were not communicated to counselors. These arenas of negotiation—the professional, public, and private—were quite separated. The different languages (Hebrew and Arabic) used by the two sides further deepened the gap.

Cousin Marriage and Carrier Matching

While many Bedouin agreed that consanguinity, and cousin marriage in particular, was responsible for the prevalence of genetic diseases, they continued to practice it. Consanguinity therefore emerges from this study as an intricate and persistent phenomenon. This is true for the Bedouin as well as for many other ethnic and traditional communities. It appears that genetics education and counseling alone are not capable of changing the pattern of consanguinity. This is particularly true in the case of relatively non-severe genetic disorders such as congenital hearing loss. The data therefore support the genetic counselors' decision to opt for "healthy consanguinity," namely carrier matching, as the focus of the genetics program.

The health professionals expected the focus on carrier matching and "healthy consanguinity" to provide for Bedouin norms and values. They also anticipated, based on their many years of experience with the Bedouin community, that carrier matching will be used in creative ways. The findings showed how genetic counseling became a multi-faceted context for negotiation. These negotiations occurred largely in the backstage, within individual, family and community contexts, rather than in the session itself. The source of the genetic disease and the proper means of prevention were negotiated and debated between health professionals and lay people, men and women, older and younger generation, high ranking and low ranking families. Interviews showed that the accounts of seed and soil (agnatic heredity), breast-feeding and 'strong eye' (uterine heredity), as well as consanguinity (Mendelian heredity) could all be used interchangeably, according to the situation and the interests of the speakers. These accounts could not be judged simply on the basis of ignorance (false) versus knowledge (true). Those who understood the medical explanation did not necessarily act on it. Educated Bedouin men, for example, who presented knowledge and positive attitudes in interviews, also had daughters that needed to be married.

Rather than being affixed to some "essential" Bedouin cultural identity, the accounts that people used for explaining the source of the disease and its preferred mode of prevention were part of a discursive, negotiated order. The medical account of heredity was indeed assimilated by many Bedouin. However, it did not simply replace other local narratives. Rather, it was used in various ways by different people so as to be challenged, modified, and sometimes merged with other, local accounts. These agendas were further reflected in the unexpected patterns of utilization that characterized some of the Bedouin. Using genetic counseling for goals such as coerced individual/stepwise testing, "wife screening" and "match breaking" was an unintended yet very real consequence of the program.

We probably understand too little of how most marriages come about to make any valid assumptions about the effect of genetic information on choice of partner. There are now several studies that support this conclusion. In Greece, where 20% of the population carry either thalassemia or sickle cell trait, all young people of marriageable age were screened and counseled in a particular study, and counseling contact was maintained for a two-year period. When the pattern of marriages was assessed at the end of this period, screening had had no measurable effect on choice of partner (Stamatoyannopoulos, 1974). In the same period a similar approach was tried in Cyprus, with the addition that marriages between carriers were actively discouraged. This proved unacceptable to the population (Angastiniotis and Hadjiminas, 1981). 98% of couples at risk detected prior to marriage proceeded to marry. Nevertheless, the annual number of new births of thalassemic children has fallen almost to zero in Cyprus. Less than 5% of this fall is due to separation of engaged couples, about 80% is due to prenatal diagnosis and selective abortion, and around 20% is because couples at risk have rather fewer children than couples not at risk (Angastiniotis et al., 1985).

In Canada, a program of information and screening for carriers of Tay-Sachs disease or thalassemia in high schools in Montreal has proved highly acceptable, and is also informative about pitfalls in predicting how people will use genetic information (Zeesman et al., 1984). A sample of the young people screened was followed up with a questionnaire that included the questions, "Do you think that a couple planning to marry who found they were both carriers would change their marriage plans? Would you change your own marriage plans?" Interestingly, almost 80% thought that other couples would change their marriage plans, but only 10% said they would change their own plans. Clearly, it is all too easy to underestimate the importance of other people's inner lives, and practical experience is the only reliable guide to how people are prepared to use information on genetic risk. On the other hand, voluntary carrier screening (among high-school students) and reproductive counseling for Tay-Sachs disease and beta-thalassemia, which have been carried out in Quebec for more than 20 years, have proven highly successful. Normal fertility rates were maintained in the families at risk, while incidence of these two diseases declined by >90% in the communities (Mitchell et al., 1996). Thus, on the one hand there seems to be a strong case for early carrier diagnosis and genetic counseling so that couples at genetic risk and their families can make an informed choice whether to separate or stay together. On the other hand, knowledge of genetic risk may be insufficient to change one of the most significant of all human decisions, choice of a marital partner.

Although all the programs summarized above showed little effect of premarital screening on the frequency of at-risk marriages, results may differ in societies with a different social and family structure, especially if a directive approach is adopted in genetic counseling. This study forcefully illustrates, however, the significance of cross-cultural training in both curricular and fieldwork activities for genetic counselors and other health professionals working with diverse ethno-cultural communities.

The Jewish-Bedouin Situation

Relations between Israeli authorities and the Bedouin are pre-determined to a large extent by prejudice and group position. The Bedouin "failure" to follow the process of sedenterization and relocation as prescribed by Israel was regarded by state officials with contempt: "The Bedouin have progressed 1,000 years during the 35 years of the Israeli rule," "they are not capable of organizing themselves" (Israeli officials cited in Jakubovska, 1990: 91). More recently, in an interview in the magazine "the Jewish Week" (July 20, 2001), Moshe Shohat, head of the Israeli Educational Authority for The Bedouin, referred to the Bedouin as "blood-thirsty people who commit polygamy, have 30 children and continue to expand their illegal settlements, taking over state land." Despite outraged reactions, Shohat retained his official position.

In sociological perspective, prejudice involves—more than negative stereotypes and negative feelings—a commitment to a relative status positioning of groups in an ethnic social order (Blumer, 1955, 1958). Such status positioning is reflected by the above-mentioned quotes from Israeli officials. It is also reflected in the rank order of the professional staff in the program. While the two certified counselors were Jewish, the four non-certified personnel were either Arab-Israeli or Bedouin.

This reality reflected existing ethnic gaps between Israeli-Jews, Israeli-Arabs and Israeli-Bedouin, but it also mirrored the sincere efforts of the Jewish health professionals who oversaw the project to tackle these ethnic gaps. An important activity of the Jewish health professionals and counselors was to train Bedouins as genetic counselors. As formal training requires several years and a bachelor degree in life sciences, it was not easy to find an adequate candidate. Nor was it easy to find the funds for the formal training. The first attempt ended with the person in training quitting for religious reasons (as described in the section entitled "The Point-of-View of Bedouin Health Professionals" in chapter three).

We also have to consider the program as an interface between the dominant Jewish medical establishment and a marginal minority—the Bedouin. There is ample literature on ethnicity and health care that focuses on the 'special needs' of members of ethnic minorities (e.g., Hahn, 1999) and the measures required to bridge the gap. This framing could also be relevant to the under-utilization of the program. Rapp (1998) similarly found that class-associated differences loomed large in explaining the variance in prenatal testing utilization. For example, middle-class patients (disproportionately White) in New York City usually accepted amniocentesis, while poorer women (disproportionately from ethnic-racial minorities) were more likely to refuse it. The question of under-utilization, however, remains open in the context of the program discussed here, since many of those tested at childhood could still return for counseling in the future.

Even if it is true that the program took place within a pre-existing framework of social order, can we safely say that counselors were prejudiced against their Bedouin customers? Counselors shared a sense of proprietary claim over their professional status. They considered themselves, in a parallel manner to physicians, not as "service providers" but as "professionals" whose higher status endows them with authority. In addition, the Jewish counselors looked at consanguinity and polygyny as traditional norms characteristic of ethnic groups that had an intrinsically different and backward culture. Nevertheless, in order to retain what was left of their nondirectiveness, counselors refrained from speaking against these norms and offered the program for premarital decisions that promoted, in their words, "healthy consanguinity." To the outsider, such an attitude might be seen as paternalistic. For the counselors, this attitude was the pragmatic outcome of many years of working with the Bedouin. Some Bedouin were also prejudiced against the program, which they saw as an extension of the dominant Israeli establishment. The program was interpreted by some, for example, as an attempt to reduce the birth rate in the Bedouin population. Under-utilization of health care services among the Bedouin in general is sometimes related to their marginal position as an ethnic, religious and political minority (Jakubowska, 1990; Shamir, 1996). This self-positioning against the "Israeli other" could have caused some Bedouin to refrain from using the program. In addition, the whole circumstances of constraint and opposition between Bedouin Arabs and Israeli identities in the Negev may have contributed to Islamization and Arabization within the Bedouin community. However, the data do not offer explicit support for this possibility.

Speaking of Agendas

One of the central issues in this study, as well as in the study of health care in general, was the issue of agendas. By bringing in the agendas of community members, this study showed that the "patients" are not necessarily passive. This was demonstrated, for example, through the story of Ā'ref, who did not marry his cousin even when the test result showed compatibility, or through the story of the Bedouin father who did not want to expose his daughter to labeling. These individual agendas were not disclosed in counseling and could be uncovered only through personal interviews with counselees. While the program for carrier matching represented a process of medicalization, this process was not unidirectional or all encompassing.

The mismatch between goals, means and results is not surprising since traditional forms of public participation that characterize the Bedouin are not conducive to Western-style 'community engagement.' Public meetings, focus groups and advisory committees impose social dynamics that are quite foreign to the Bedouin. These forums do not comprise the actual social channels of communication and decision-making. The findings show that men who participated in public meetings generally supported the program. Such a statement could also reflect the socially appropriate sentiment in public contexts, in which members emphasize the interests of the community as a whole (cf. Foster et al., 1998; Andrews, 1994). In individual interviews, such support was not a matter of consensus. Instead, individuals used or rejected the program according to personal interests.

The mismatch between private and public arenas of negotiation is very clear in the context of Bedouin women. Women live in a sub-society, which is both separate from and parallel to the men's (Abu-Lughod, 1985). Their agendas were not expressed in public meetings since they were not present there. In almost all the cases, it was a Bedouin man who came for counseling. The utilization of the program by men demonstrated a patriarchal status system. However, the examples presented here do not mean that the program could not fulfill its mission for some counselees. What they do show us, in general, is that counseling does not occur in a vacuum. When used, it always becomes entangled in people's lives, and their interests and constraints shape its outcomes. To date, policy frameworks for genetic counseling have focused on perceived benefits and risks of the individual. Yet the individual level, which concerns the patient-counselor interaction, often also depends on community-level norms.

A mismatch in agendas has also been demonstrated by Bosk's (1992) observation in relation to pediatric genetic counseling services in the US. He states that:

> "To borrow from Merton (1957), if genetic counselors are cosmopolitan when understanding genetic disease, patients are locals. In everyday terms, this means that genetic counselors' explanations are framed in universal terms. They are valid not just for the current couple receiving counseling, but for all patients in this disease category. Explanations are focused on abstract, impersonal, biological processes. Conversely, parent understandings are very specific and personal. They are fashioned out of highly situated understandings for this particular pregnancy, this particular family, this particular person" (Bosk, 1992: 48).

The "cosmopolitans versus locals" distinction, arguably a general phenomenon built into the counseling process, can be said to be even more evident in the case studied here. The counselors working with the Bedouin community were "cosmopolitans" not only in Bosk's sense of framing their explanations in universal terms, but also in the sense of representing a global biomedical culture. Their cosmopolitan characteristics were indeed accentuated (and thus also required moderation and cultural adaptation) by the clearly 'local' characteristics of the counselees, namely the traditional norms of Bedouin culture. It can hardly be expected that common agendas will emerge from such a situation in the short run. What this study has shown us is a gradual, perhaps ungainly and awkward process of glocalization and hybridization. The intricate and multi-faceted negotiated order of community genetics, as manifested in this study, evades (indeed defies) broader and perhaps more captivating definitions of either modernization or medicalization. Nevertheless, it is through such negotiations, clumsy and hybrid as they may appear to the Western observer, that social reality is constructed.

Communitarian and Liberal Perspectives on Community Genetics

In the US and Europe, the trend in human genetics has been towards a development of universal and standard criteria such as informed consent, nondirectiveness, and autonomy (e.g., reproductive freedom). Chadwick (1998:

474) calls this the "standard view" of genetic counseling. This view generally means moving away from "community genetics" as a concept implying cultural relativity. However, this study showed that the concepts of nondirectiveness and autonomy depend on communal norms of interpretation. Bedouin individuals, particularly women, are often not "autonomous" but depend on others, and reproductive "freedom" is limited by community expectations and religious bans.

The dilemmas of community genetics can be framed within the communitarian-liberal debate (Strike 2000; Watson 1999). Scholars like Alasdair MacIntyre, Michael Sandel, Charles Taylor, Amitai Etzioni and Michael Walzer, who have led the recent communitarian renaissance in the US, have argued that moral life is rooted in the norms of particular communities. Liberalism, in contrast, has sought for norms that are universal and generalizable (similar to the conception of the "standard view" in genetic counseling). While liberals argue that communitarianism is likely to be parochial and sectarian, communitarians claim that liberalism is a "view from nowhere" that is more likely to produce rootlessness and anomie than justice.

The norms of the Bedouin community are underpinned by kinship and religion to an extent no longer characteristic of modern, Western countries. This situation, however, is characteristic of many developing countries as well as immigrant communities. In these societies, values such as authority, obligation, honor and caring are family-centered. In contrast, the focus of Western bioethics is on the individual (Beauchamp, 1997). Following this logic, it can be argued that different cultures produce and require different forms of bioethics. Although physicians around the world are concerned with healing diseases and help their patients, such concerns are already shaped by religious, moral, and cultural values. Medical interactions are situated within social expectations and treatment obligations. Tan Alora and Lumitao (2001) have recently shown that in the Philippines, North American bioethical standards are often at odds with a culture in which family relationships take precedence over individualism. For example, truth-telling is accorded not to the patient but to his or her family, and consent forms are either signed by the senior family member or regarded as irrelevant because of the paternalistic context of physician-patient relationship. Based on the Filipino case, which shares many similarities with that of the Bedouin, Tan Alora and Lumitao propose a meta-ethical thesis regarding the incommensurability of North American and Filipino bioethics (see also Hoshino, 1997). In their view,

> "The Western moral principles of autonomy, beneficence, non-malficence, and justice contrast with Filipino moral concerns; from the

Filipino perspective, the former are starkly individualistic, atomistic, and marked by a degree of anomie."

Accounting for the cultural differences that underlie such global-local intersections, however important, is not enough. Moral vocabularies and ethical grammars, however elaborate, cannot predict what is actually going to take place in the medical interaction and as a result of it. Decision-making and utilization are always realized within the flow of an interactive and negotiated order. While underpinned by Muslim and collectivist premises, Bedouin agendas are also determined by political circumstances as well as personal interests.

In considering the practical implications of this study, the dilemma for health professionals and those interested in community genetics is whether to remain loyal to the standard bioethical view of non-directiveness (which according to my findings is probably misinterpreted in any event), or to be directive for the sake of medical efficiency, as many of the Bedouin respondents indeed suggested. This dilemma is not unique to the Bedouin context and the program for carrier matching studied here. It is characteristic of many other health care contexts and, indeed, relevant to counseling in general. While my findings have hopefully helped to sharpen the dilemma and clarify its implications for the negotiated order of the carrier matching program, in the final analysis, one's solution to this dilemma depends on one's values. Health professionals that seek to induce change in the name of biomedical modernization and to reduce the prevalence of genetic diseases in a targeted population should be directive in order to be efficient. In the same vein, health professionals who subscribe to the ideal of non-directiveness should attempt to preserve local customs for the sake of tradition. These two goals are enmeshed in the organizational culture of genetic counseling. While the value of non-directiveness constitutes an important part of the espoused theory of counselors, the goal of reducing the prevalence of genetic diseases is very likely, as this study has shown, a part of their practice and theory-in-use. According to the organizational analysts Argyris and Schon (1979), espoused theories prescribe what people say about their job, but theories-in-use explain what people are actually doing on the job. The values of non-directiveness and medical efficiency are inherently in conflict, and there is no easy way out of this conflict.

The consequences of this dilemma should also be examined in the context of the specific NSRD program studied here as well as in the general context of community-based programs for genetic counseling. In the case of the NSRD program, the need for this intervention is arguably questioned when considering the mildness of the condition tested for (congenital hearing loss). When participating in the implementation and evaluation of the NSRD program, the health professionals and I believed that NSRD would not remain the only condition tested for in the targeted community. It was indeed the intention of geneticists to add other genetic tests for severe diseases that were prevalent in the clan, as soon as the on-going genetic research would provide a reliable identification of the mutation. In general, however, community-based intervention programs for genetic counseling can be both medically needed and ethically justified. For this to happen, several criteria should be applied. In terms of medical need, the program should offer genetic testing for a condition which is life-threatening or severe enough according to both affected individuals and health professionals, with an early onset, and high probability of development in the affected individual. These criteria were discussed in the section titled "bioethical criteria for genetic screening" in chapter three. In terms of ethical justification, a process of community engagement and empowerment should take place prior to and alongside the implementation of the intervention program. This position hinges on a communitarian perspective and contrasts the liberal, universalistic perspective which is currently the "standard view" (in the US and Europe) of genetic counseling. This is why, as I argued at the outset of this book, the emerging field of "community genetics" requires the development of a new paradigm for genetic counseling.

To follow the ebb and flow of social interaction, one must first become involved in it through participant observation. Yet in order to realize the micropolitical circumstances and personal interests that converge in the agendas of participants, one must first implement a community-based intervention program. The process of working towards better understanding is therefore replete with daily struggles and mistakes. This is one reason why eliciting community needs and attitudes is so difficult in this and similar settings (Nichter, 1999). When one is walking it is difficult to see the soles of one's feet. I hope this study will join other reflexive and ethnographic accounts of community-based programs for genetic counseling in order to enrich our understanding of these complex processes and contribute to the development of a new paradigm of community genetics, of which we are greatly in need. All those involved in community-based genetic counseling, as well as other community-based medical services, should be alert to these questions and to the delicate balance of advocacy and control they invoke.

Appendix: Questionnaire Assessing the Interpretation of Counseling

First version ("pessimistic")

1. Your younger brother has Tay-Sachs. You've met a person that may become your fiancé/e. There were persons affected by Tay-Sachs in his/her family too. Both of you decide to use genetic counseling. The genetic counselor tells you: "the test shows you're both carrying the Tay-Sachs gene. It means you have 25 percent risk in each pregnancy to have an affected child. You should know this is a severe disease with no available treatment. An affected child often suffers from mental retardation and dies at young age. The test you've done is as close to 100 percent reliability as possible. There is also a prenatal Tay-Sachs test that can be done in each pregnancy."

(Questions and response options appear in tables 8–9 and are not repeated here).

2. You have come for counseling following amniocentesis. The genetic counselor tells you: "In a genetic test, whose reliability is as close to 100 percent as possible, it was found that the fetus has Down Syndrome. It is a severe disease with no available treatment. Usually there are additional problems such as heart defects, muscle weakness, and a characteristic face pattern. The major problem is mental retardation. The child is going to require care and inspection throughout his/her life."

Second version ("optimistic")

1. Your younger brother has Tay-Sachs. You've met a person that may become your fiancé/e. There were persons affected by Tay-Sachs in his/her family too. You decide to use genetic counseling. The genetic counselor tells you:

"the test shows you're both carrying the Tay-Sachs gene. It means you still have 75 percent chance in each pregnancy to have a healthy child. You should know this is a severe disease with no available treatment. An affected child often suffers from mental retardation and dies at young age. The test you've done is as close to 100 percent reliability as possible. There is also a prenatal Tay-Sachs test that can be done in each pregnancy."

2. You have come for counseling following amniocentesis. The genetic counselor tells you: "In a genetic test, whose reliability is as close to 100 percent as possible, it was found that the fetus has Down Syndrome. It is a severe disease with no available treatment. The child is going to suffer from mental retardation and require care and inspection throughout his/her life. All affected children suffer from mental retardation, however there's a spectrum—from profound to medium. We cannot tell in advance the degree of retardation. Usually there are additional problems such as heart defects, muscle weakness, and a characteristic face pattern. The major problem is mental retardation."

Glossary

Alleles: variant forms of the same gene.

Amniocentesis: until recently, the accepted mainstay of prenatal genetic diagnosis. Amniocentesis involves inserting a needle into the amniotic sac surrounding the fetus. Amniocentesis is performed between 14–16 weeks of gestation and test results take an additional two weeks.

Autosome: Any chromosome other than a sex chromosome. Humans have 22 pairs of autosomes. Hence, autosomal: belonging to a chromosome other than a sex chromosome.

Carrier: a person who has a recessive mutated gene, together with its normal allele. Carriers do not usually develop the disease but can pass the mutated gene on to their children.

Carrier testing: testing to identify individuals who carry disease-causing recessive genes that could be inherited by their children. Carrier testing is designed for healthy people who have no symptoms of disease, but who are known to be at high risk because of family history.

Congenital: any trait or condition that exists from birth.

Cystic fibrosis: an inherited disease in which thick mucus clogs the lungs and blocks the ducts of the pancreas.

Chorionic villus sampling (CVS): a relatively new procedure used to diagnose certain birth defects in the first trimester of pregnancy, between ten and twelve weeks from the first day of the last menstrual period. The procedure involves inserting a small catheter (tube) through the cervix and into the developing placenta. A bit of placental tissue is then gently suctioned into a syringe. Both the placental and fetal tissues originate from the same cell line and are genetically identical. Thus, by obtaining a tiny sample of the chorionic villi from the placenta, one can determine certain genetic characteristics of the fetus.

DNA: the substance of heredity, a large molecule that carries the genetic information that cells need to replicate and to produce proteins.

Dominant allele: a gene that is expressed, regardless of whether its counterpart allele is dominant or recessive. Autosomal dominant disorders are produced by a single mutated dominant allele.

Gene: a unit of inheritance; a working subunit of DNA. Each of the body's genes contains the code for a specific product, typically a protein.

Genome: all the genetic material in the chromosomes of a particular organism.

Heterozygous: possessing two different forms of a particular gene, one inherited from each parent.

Homozygous: possessing two identical forms of a particular gene, one inherited from each parent.

Human Genome Project: an international research effort (led in the US by the National Institutes of Health and the Department of Energy) aimed at identifying and ordering every base in the human genome.

Huntington's disease: An autosomal dominant genetic disease causing degenerative brain disorder that usually appears in mid-life. Its symptoms, which include involuntary movement of the face and limbs, mood swings, and forgetfulness, get worse as the disease progresses. It is generally fatal within 20 years.

Mutation: a permanent change in the number, arrangement or molecular sequence of a gene.

Maternal serum screening: A biochemical test for the detection of fetal genetic abnormalities (such as trisomy 21 and neural tube defects). The serum markers most widely used are alfa-fetoprotein, unconjugated estriol, and human chorionic gonadotropin. This combination is known as "triple test." The maternal serum levels of these proteins and of steroid hormones vary with the gestational age for the pregnancy. The triple test is usually performed at 15 to 18 weeks of gestation. The level of each serum marker is measured and reported as a multiple of the median for women with pregnancies of the same gestational age as that of the patient's. The likelihood of fetal genetic abnormalities is calculated on the basis of each of the serum marker results and the patient's age. A positive test is an indication for amniocentesis.

Newborn screening: examining blood samples from a newborn infant to detect disease-related abnormalities or deficiencies in gene products.

Prenatal diagnosis: examining fetal cells taken from the amniotic fluid, the primitive placenta (chorion), or the umbilical cord for chromosomal or gene alterations.

Recessive allele: a gene that is expressed only when its counterpart allele on the matching chromosome is also recessive. Autosomal recessive disorders develop in persons who receive two copies of the mutant gene, one from each parent who is a carrier.

Sickle cell anemia: an inherited, potentially lethal disease in which a defect in hemoglobin, the oxygen-carrying pigment in the blood, causes distortion (sickling) and loss of red blood cells, producing damage to organs throughout the body.

Single nucleotide polymorphism (SNP): common but minute variations that occur in human DNA. These variations can be used to track inheritance in families.

Tay-Sachs disease: an inherited disease of infancy characterized by profound mental retardation and early death; it is caused by a recessive gene mutation.

Thalassemia: a genetically determined disorder characterized by reduced production of hemoglobin chains in red blood cells, thus usually causing severe anemia.

Source: National Human Genome Research Institute, National Institutes of Health (2000) "Glossary of Genetic Terms." Information is available at http://www.genome.gov/glossary.cfm.

References Cited

Abd al-Ati, Hammudah (1995). *The Family Structure in Islam.* Plainfield-Indiana: American Trust Publications. First published in 1977.

Abeliovich D, Quint A, Weinberg N, Verchezon G, Lerer I, Eckstein J, Rubinstein E. (1996). "Cystic Fibrosis Heterozygote screening in the orthodox community of Ashkenazi Jews: The Dor Yesharim approach and heterozygote frequency." *European Journal of Human Genetics* 4: 77–82.

Abu-Lughod, L. (1986). *Veiled Sentiments: Honor and Poetry in a Bedouin Society.* Berkeley: University of California Press.

————. (1985). "A Community of Secrets: The Separate World of Bedouin Women." *Signs* 10(4): 637–57.

Abu-Rabi'a A'ref. (1983). "Traditional medicine among the Bedouin tribes of the Negev." *Notes on the Bedouins* 14: 341–57 (Hebrew).

————. (1999). *Traditional Bedouin Medicine.* Ministry of Defense Publications Office (Hebrew).

————. (2000). "Employment and Unemployment among the Negev Bedouin," *Nomadic Peoples* 4(2): 84–93.

Ahmad, W., Darr, A., Johnes, L. & Nisar, G. (1998). *Deafness and Ethnicity: Services, Policy and Politics.* Bristol: Policy Press.

Anderson, Benedict. (1983). *Imagined Communities.* London: Verso.

Andrews, L. (1994). "Public Choices and Private Choices: Legal Regulation of Genetic Testing." In Murphy, T. & M. Lappé (eds.) *Justice and the Human Genome Project.* Berkeley: U of California Press, pp. 46–75.

Angastiniotis MA, Hadjiminas MG. (1981). "Prevention of thalassemia in Cyprus." *Lancet,* 1: 369–70.

Angastiniotis MA, Kyriakidou S, Hadjiminas M. (1986). "How thalassemia was controlled in Cyprus." *World health forum,* 7: 291–97.

Annual statistics for 1998. Central Bureau of Statistics, Israel.

Argyris, C. & D. Schon (1979). *Organizational Learning.* NY: Addison-Wesley

Arnos, K, Israel, J. & M. Cunningham (1991). "Genetic counseling for the deaf: Medical and cultural considerations." *Journal of Genetic Counseling* 630: 212–22.

Asad, T. (1986). "The concept of cultural translation in British social anthropology." In Clifford, J. & G. Marcus (Eds.) *Writing Culture: The Poetics and Politics of Ethnography.* Berkeley: University of California Press. Pp. 141–64.

Asali, Abed, Khamaysi, Naif, Aburabia, Yunis, Letzer, Simha, et al. (1995). "Ritual female genital surgery among Bedouin in Israel," *Archives of Sexual Behavior* 24(5): 571–80.

Atkin, K., Ahmad, W., & L. Jones (2002). "Young south Asian deaf people and their families: negotiating relationships and identities." *Sociology of Health and Illness* 24(1): 21–45.

Azaiza, Faisal (1996). "Family Planning among Rural Moslem Women in Israel," *Journal of Comparative Family Studies* 27(3): 559–68.

Barry, Christine, Bradley, Colin, Britten, Nicky, Stevenson, Fiona & Barber, Nick (2000). "Patients' unvoiced agendas in general practice consultations: qualitative study." *British Medical Journal*, 320(7244): 1246–51.

Baudrillard, Jean. (1983). *Simulations.* NY: Semiotext(e).

———. (1988). *The Ecstasy of Communication.* NY: Semiotext.

Beauchamp, T. & J. Childress (1994). *Principles of Biomedical Ethics.* NY: Oxford UP.

Beauchamp, T. (1997). "Comparative Studies: Japan and America." In *Japanese and Western Bioethics*, K. Hoshino (ed.). Kluwer Academic Press, pp. 25–48.

Beckerleg, S. et al. (1997). "Eliciting Local Voices Using Natural Group Interviews," *Anthropology & Medicine* 4(3): 273–88.

Berkenstadt, M., Shiloh, S., Barkai, G., Katzenelson, M., Goldman, B. (1999). "Perceived personal control (PPC): a new concept in measuring outcome in genetic counseling." *American Journal of Medical Genetics* 82: 53–59.

Bienvenu, M. & B. Colonomus. 1985. *An Introduction to American Deaf Culture.* Silver Spring, MD: Sign Media.

Bittles, Alan H. (1994). "The role and significance of consanguinity as a demographic variable." *Population and development review*, 20: 561–83.

———. (1992). "Consanguinity: a major variable in studies on North African reproductive behaviour, morbidity and mortality?" In: Moore S, ed. *Proceedings of the demographic and health surveys world conference.* Columbia, MD, Macro International, 1: 321–41.

Bittles, Alan H. et al. (1991). "Reproductive behaviour and health in consanguineous marriages." *Science*, 252: 789–94.

Bleiker, E. Aaronson, A., Menko, F. (1997). "Genetic counseling for hereditary cancer: A pilot of experiences of family members." *Patient Education and Counseling* 32: 107–16.

Blumer, Herbert. (1955). "Reflections on theory of race relations." In A. W. Lind (ed.), *Race relations in world perspective* (pp. 3–21). Honolulu: University of Hawaii Press.

————. (1958). "Race prejudice as a sense of group position." *Pacific Sociological Review*, I, 3–7.

Bobo, L. (1999). "Prejudice as Group Position: Microfoundations of a Sociological Approach to Racism and Race Relations." *Journal of Social Issues*, 55(3): 445–54.

Borkan, J., M. Morad & S. Shvarts (2000). "Universal Health Care? The views of Negev Bedouin Arabs on health services," *Health Policy and Planning* 15(2): 207–16

Bosk, Charles. (1992). *All God's Mistakes: Genetic Counseling in a Pediatric Hospital.* Chicago: University of Chicago Press.

Boss, J. (1993). *The Birth Lottery, Prenatal Diagnosis and Selective Abortion.* Chicago: Loyola University Press.

Brisson, D. (2000). "Analysis and integration of definitions of community genetics," *Community Genetics* 3: 99–101.

Broad, C. (1930). *Five Types of Ethical Theory.* London: Kegan and Paul.

Britton, B. & A. Pellegrini (1991). *Narrative Thought and Narrative Language.* Hillsdale, NJ: Lawrence Erlbaum Associates.

Broide E, Zeigler M, Eckstein J, Bach G. (1993). "Screening for carriers of Tay-Sachs disease in the ultraorthodox Ashkenazi Jewish community in Israel." *American Journal of Medical Genetics* 47: 21–35.

Burke, B. & A. Kolker (1994). "Directiveness in Prenatal Genetic Counseling." *Women and Health* 22: 31–53.

Cantor RM, Novak JM, Bass EN, Crandall BF. (1997). "PCR-based screening for cystic fibrosis carrier mutations in an ethnically diverse pregnant population." *American Journal of Human Genetics* 60: 935–47.

Cao A, Saba L. Galanello R, Rosatelli MC. (1997). "Molecular diagnosis and carrier screening for beta thalassemia." *JAMA* 278: 1273–77.

Caplan, A. M. Glenn & D. Magnus (1999). "What is immoral about eugenics?" *British Medical Journal*, 319(7220): 1284–87.

Carmi, R., Elbedour K., D. Weitzman, V. Sheffield & I. Shoham-Vardi (1998). "Lowering the Burden of Hereditary Diseases in a Traditional Inbred Community: Ethical Aspects of Genetic Research and its Application." *Science in Context* 11(3–4): 391–95.

Carmi R, Elbedour K, Stone EM, Sheffield V. (1995). "Phenotype differences among patients with Bardet-Biedl syndrome linked to different chromosome loci." *American Journal of Medical Genetics* 59: 199–203.

Chadwick, Ruth. (1998). "Can Genetic Counseling Avoid the Charge of Eugenics?" *Science in Context* 11(3–4): 471–81.

Chadwick, Ruth. et al. (1999). *The Ethics of Genetic Screening.* Dordrecht: Kluwer.

Chapple, A. & C. May (1996). "Genetic knowledge and family relationships: two case studies." *Health and Social Care in the Community* 4(3): 166–71.

Chapple, A., Campion, P. & C. May (1997). "Clinical terminology: anxiety and confusion amongst families undergoing genetic counseling." *Patient Education and Counseling* 32: 81–91.

Christakis N. (1992). "Ethics are local: Engaging cross-cultural variation in the ethics for clinical research." *Socical Science & Medicine* 35: 1079–91.

Clarke, Angus. (1991). "Is non-directive genetic counselling possible?" (editorial) *The Lancet*, 338(8773): 998(4).

Clarke, Angus & Evelyn Parsons (Eds.) (1996). *Culture, Kinship and Genes: Towards Cross-Cultural Genetics.* London: MacMillan Press.

Clifford, James. (1990). "Notes on (Field)notes." In R. Sanjek (ed.), *Fieldnotes: The making of anthropology.* Ithaca: Cornell University Press, pp. 47–71.

Cohen, Jacob. (1969). *Statistical Power Analysis for the Social Sciences.* NY: Academic Press.

Cohn, E., P. Kelley, T. Fowler, M. Gorga et al. (1999). "Clinical studies of families with hearing loss attributable to mutations in the Connexin 26 gene (GJB2/DFNB1)," *Pediatrics* 103(3): 546–50.

Cohen, M. & R. Gorlin (1995). "Epidemiology, etiology and genetic patterns." In: Gorlin R. Toriello H, Cohen M. (Eds.) *Hereditary Hearing Loss and Its Syndromes.* Oxford: Oxford University Press, pp. 9–21.

Comaroff, John & Jean Comaroff. (1997). *Of Revelation and Revolution*, Chicago IL: University of Chicago Press.

——————— (eds.) (1992). *Ethnography and the Historical Imagination.* Boulder: Westview Press.

Comaroff, Jean. (1992). "Bodily reform as historical practice." In Comaroff, J. & J. Comaroff (eds.) *Ethnography and the Historical Imagination.* Boulder: Westview Press. Pp. 69–91.

Conrad, Peter. (1975). "The discovery of hyperkinesis: Notes on the medicalization of deviant behavior." *Social Problems* 23: 12–21.

———. (1992). "Medicalization and social control." *Annual Review of Sociology* 18: 209–32.

———. (1997). "Public eyes and private genes: historical frames, news constructions, and social problems." *Social Problems* 44: 139–54.

———. (1999) "A mirage of genes." *Sociology of Health and Illness* 21(2): 228–39.

Conrad, Peter & Jonathan Gabe (Eds.) (1999). *Sociological Perspectives on the New Genetics.* Oxford: Blackwell's.

Cuckle, H. & Wald, N. (1994). "Principles of Screening." In Wald, N. (ed.) *Antenatal and Neonatal Screening.* Oxford: Oxford UP.

Darr, Aamra. (1997). "Consanguineous marriage and genetics: a positive relationship." Pp. 83–97 in Angus Clarke and Evelyn Parsons (Eds.), *Culture, Kinship and Genes.* London: MacMillan Press.

———. (1990). The social aspects of thalassemia major among Muslims of Pakistani origin in England: family experience and service delivery. PhD thesis, University College, London.

Davidov, B. et al (1994). "Prenatal testing for Down syndrome in the Jewish and non-Jewish populations in Israel." *Israel Journal of Medical Sciences* 30: 629–33.

Davis D. (2001). *Genetic Dilemmas: Reproductive Technology, Parental Choices, and Children's Futures.* London: Routledge.

Davis, John (1977). *Peoples of the Mediterranean.* London: Routledge.

Delaney, Carol. (1991). *The Seed and the Soil: Gender and Cosmology in Turkish Village Society.* Berkeley: University of California Press.

Denzin, Norman. (1978). *The Research Act.* NY: Aldine.

Dinero, Steven (1998). "Social Adaptation and Welfare Planning in the Post-Nomadic Urban Environment: The Case of the Israeli Negev Bedouin," *Journal of Community Practice* 5(3): 15–36.

———. (1997). "Female role change and male response in the post-nomadic urban environment: The case of the Israeli Negev Bedouin." *Journal of Comparative Family Studies* 28(3): 248–61.

Drlica, K. (1994). *Double-Edged Sword: the Promises and Risks of the Genetic Revolution.* Reading, MA: Addison-Wesley Publishing Company.

Dunne, C. and C. Warren. (1998). "Lethal autonomy: the malfunction of the informed consent mechanism within the context of prenatal diagnosis of genetic variants." *Issues in Law & Medicine,* 14,2: 165–81.

Eunpu, D. (1997). "Systematically-based psychotherapeutic techniques in genetic counseling." *Journal of Genetic Counseling* 6: 1–20.

Falk, Raphael (1998). "Zionism and the Biology of the Jews," *Science in Context* 11(3–4): 587–607.

Farrell, M. L. Certain & P. Farrell (2001). "Genetic Counseling and Risk Communication Services of Newborn Screening Programs." *Archives of Pediatrics & Adolescent Medicine*, 155(2): 120–41.

Fedida, Michael. (1984). Honor, kinship and marriage in Arab culture. PhD dissertation, U of Chicago, Ill.

Fish, Stanley. (1980). *Is There a Text in This Class?—The Authority of Interpretive Communities.* Harvard: Harvard UP.

Fraser F. (1974). "Genetic counseling." *American Journal of Human Genetics* 26: 636–59.

Foster, M., Eisenbraun AJ, Carter TH. (1998). "Genetic screening of targeted subpopulations: use of communal discourse to evaluate sociocultural implications." *Genetic Screening* 1(4): 269–74.

Freundlich, E & N. Hino. (1984). "Consanguineous marriage among rural Arabs in Israel." *Israel Journal of Medical Sciences* 20: 1035–38.

Fried K, Davies AM. (1974). "Some effects on the offspring of uncle-niece marriage in the Moroccan Jewish community in Jerusalem." *American journal of human genetics*, 26: 65–72.

Gerhardt, Uta. (2000). "Ambivalent Interactionist: Anselm Strauss and the "Schools" of Chicago Sociology." *American Sociologist*, 31(4): 34–71.

Gilbar, G. (1997). *Population dilemmas in the Middle East.* London: Frank Cass.

Groce, Nora. (1985). *Everyone Here Spoke Sign Language: Hereditary Deafness on Martha's Vineyard.* Cambridge, MA: Harvard University Press.

Hadjiminas, Minas (1994). The Cyprus Experience—screening to combat a serious genetic disease. Proceedings of the 2nd symposium of the Council of Europe on Bioethics, Strasbourg, 30 Nov – 2 Dec 1993.

Hahn, R. (ed.) (1999). *Anthropology in Public Health.* Oxford: Oxford UP.

Haldane, J.B.S. (1963). "The implications of genetics for human society." In: Geerts SJ, ed. *Genetics today: proceedings of the 11th international congress of human genetics.* The Hague, Pergamon Press, pp. 91–102.

Hand, W. (1980). "Deformity, disease, and physical ailment as divine retribution." In *Magical Medicine.* Berkeley: University of California Press, pp. 57–67.

Hannerz, Ulf. (1992). *Cultural Complexity.* New York: Columbia University Press.

————. (1996). *Transnational Connections.* London: Routledge.

Hazan, H. (2000). *Simulated Dreams: Israeli Youth and Zionism*. London: Berghan Press.

Have, H. ten, & G. Kimsma (1990). "Changing Conception s of Medical Ethics," in: U. Jensen & G. Mooney (Eds.) *Changing Values in medical and Health-Care Decision Making*, Chichester: Wiley & Sons, pp. 33–51.

Henneman, L., I. Bramsen; H. M. van der Ploeg; H J Ader; H E van der Horst; J J P Gille; L P ten Kate (2001). "Participation in preconceptional carrier couple screening: characteristics, attitudes, and knowledge of both partners." *Journal of Medical Genetics*, 38(10): 695–707.

Hildes, E., Jacobs, H., Cameron, A. (1993). "Impact of genetic counseling after neonatal screening for Duchenne Muscular Dystrophy." *Journal of Medical Genetics* 30: 670–74.

Hoedemaeker, Rogeer. (1998). *Normative Determinants of Genetic Screening and testing*. Wageningen: Ponsen en Looijen.

———————. (1999). "Genetic screening and testing: a moral map." Pp. 207–30 in R. Chadwick et al. (eds.), *The Ethics of Genetic Screening*. Dodrecht: Kluwer.

Hoedemaeker, Rogeer & Henk ten Have (1998). "Geneticization: The Cyprus Case." *Journal of Medicine and Philosophy* 23(3): 274–87.

Holtzman, N., D. Shapiro (1998). "Genetic testing and public policy," *British Medical Journal* 316(7134): 852–55.

Holzgreve, W. E. Sevinchan, E. Kohne, S. Sevinchan, P. Miny & J. Horst (1990). "Beta-Thalassemia problems in the Turkish population in the F.R.G." *European Journal of Obstetrics & Gynecology and Reproductive Biology* 34: 137–47.

Honnor M, Zubrick SR, Walpole I, Bower C, Goldblatt J. (2000). "Population screening for cystic fibrosis in Western Australia: community response." *American Journal of Medical Genetics* 93: 198–204.

Hoshino, K. (ed.) (1997). *Japanese and Western Bioethics: Studies in Moral Diversity*. Dodrecht: Kluwer.

Illich, I. (1976). *Medical Nemesis*. New York: Pantheon.

Institute of Medicine. (1994). Assessing Genetic Risks: Implications for Health and Social Policy. Washington: National Academy Press.

Ioannou, Panayiotis (1999). "Thalassemia prevention in Cyprus." Pp. 55–67 in R. Chadwick et al. (eds.), *The Ethics of Genetic Screening*. Dodrecht: Kluwer.

Israel, J. et al. (1992). "Genetic counseling for deaf adults: communications/language and cultural considerations." *Journal of Genetic Counseling* 1(2): 135–52.

Jakubovska, L. (1990). "Resisting 'Ethnicity': The Israeli State and Bedouin Identity," pp. 85–105 in Nordstrom, C. & J. Martin (Eds.), *The Paths to Domination, Resistance and Terror,* Berkeley: University of California Press.

Johnson, S. (1990). "Toward clarifying culture, race, and ethnicity in the context of multicultural counseling." *Journal of Multicultural Counseling Development* 18: 41–50.

Kaback MM, Becker ME, Ruth MV. (1974) "Sociological studies in human genetics. I. Compliance factors in a voluntary heterozygote screening program." *Birth Defects,* 10: 145–63.

Kahn, Susan (2000). *Reproducing Jews: A Cultural Account of Assisted Conception in Israel.* Durham: Duke University Pres.

Katriel, Tamar (1986). *Talking Straight: Dugri Speech in Israeli Sabra Culture.* Cambridge: Cambridge University Press.

Kelly, T. (1986). *Clinical genetics and Genetic Counseling.* Chicago: Year Book.

Kanaaneh, Rhoda Ann. (2002). *Birthing the Nation: Strategies of Palestinian Women in Israel.* Berkeley and Los Angeles, CA: University of California Press.

Kessler S. (1992a). "Psychological aspects of genetic counseling VII: Thoughts on directiveness." *Journal of Genetic Counseling* 1: 9–17.

———. (1992b). "Process issues in genetic counseling." *Birth Defects* 28(1): 1–10.

Kessler, S. (1997). "Psychological aspects of genetic counseling XI: Nondirectiveness revisited." *American Journal of Medical Genetics* 72: 164–71.

Kessler, S. & Bloch, M. (1989). "Social system response to Huntington Disease." *Family Process* 28: 59–68.

Kerr, Anne, Sarah Cunningham-Burley and Amanda Amos. (1998). "Eugenics and the new genetics in Britain: examining contemporary professionals' accounts." *Science, Technology & Human Values,* 23(2): 175–99.

Khlat, M., Khudr A. (1986). "Cousin marriages in Beirut, Lebanon: is the pattern changing?" *Journal of biosocial science* 16: 369–73.

Khlat, M. (1988). "Consanguineous marriage and reproduction in Beirut, Lebanon." *American journal of human genetics,* 43: 188–96.

Khoury MJ, Burke W, Thomson EJ (eds) (2000). *Genetics and public health in the 21st century: Using genetic information to improve health and prevent disease.* Oxford: Oxford University Press.

Khuri FI. (1970). "Parallel cousin marriage considered: A Middle Eastern practice that nullifies the effects of marriage on the intensity of family relationships". *Man* 4: 597–618.

Kirscht, J.P. (1988). "The health belief model and predictions of health actions." In Gochman D.S. (ed), *Health behavior: Emerging research perspectives.* New York: Plenum Press, pp. 27–42.

Kisch, Shifra (2000). "Deaf discourse: The social construction of deafness in a Bedouin community." MA thesis, Tel-Aviv University, Israel (Hebrew).

Knoppers, B. (2000). "From Medical Ethics to 'Genethics'," *The Lancet* 356: S38.

King, P. (1992). "The past as prologue: race, class, and gene discrimination." In Annas G. & Elias, S. (eds). *Gene Mapping: using law and ethics as guides.* Oxford: Oxford University Press, pp. 94–111.

Krawczak, M., D. Cooper & J. Schmidtke. (2001). "Estimating the Efficacy and Efficiency of Cascade Genetic Screening." *American Journal of Human Genetics,* 69(2): 361–92.

Kressel, Gideon (1986). "Prescriptive patrilateral parallel cousin marriage: The perspective of the bride's father and brothers." *Ethnology* 25: 163–80.

————. (1992). *Descent through Males.* Harrassowitz, Wiesbaden.

————. (1992a) "Shame and Gender." *Anthropological Quarterly* 65(1): 34–46.

Ladd, P. (1990). "Making plans for Nigel: The erosion of identity by mainstreaming." In: Taylor, G., & Bishop, J. (Eds.) *Being Deaf: the experience of deafness.* London: Pinter.

————. (1991). "The modern deaf community." In Gregory, S., & Hartley, G. (eds.) *Constructing Deafness.* London: Pinter.

Laqueur, Walter (1972). *A History of Zionism.* NY: Basic Books.

Lavie, Smadar. (1990). *The Poetics of Military Occupation.* Berkeley: University of California Press.

Lerman, C. Scwartz, M. Lin T., Hughes C., Narod S., Lynch H. (1997). "The influence of psychological distress on use of genetic testing for cancer risk." *Journal of Counseling and Clinical Psychology* 65: 414–20.

Lewando-Hundt, G., I. Shoham-Vardi, I. Beckerelg, I. Belmaker, F. Kassem and A. Abu Jaafar (2001). "Knowledge, Action and Resistance: The Selective Use of Prenatal Screening Among Bedouin Women of the Negev, Israel." *Social Science and Medicine* 52: 561–69.

Lim Tan, M. (1989). "Traditional or transitional medical systems? Pharmacotherapy as a case for analysis." *Social Science and Medicine* 29(3): 301–7.

Lippman, Amy (1992). "Led (Astray) by Genetic Maps: The cartography of the Human Genome and health care," *Social Science and Medicine* 35: 1469–76.

Lock, M. (1998). "Perfecting Society: Reproductive Technologies, Genetic Testing, and The Planned Family in Japan." In M. Lock and P. Kaufert,

Pragmatic Women and Body Politics. Pp. 206–39. Cambridge: Cambridge University Press.

Marks, E. (1974). *The Bedouin society in the Negev.* Tel-Aviv, Israel: Reshafim Press (in Hebrew).

Marks, E. (2000). "Land and work: Negev Bedouin struggle with Israeli bureaucracies." *Nomadic Peoples,* 4(2): 106–22

McKusick, V. (1990). *Mendelian Inheritance in Man.* Baltimore: Johns Hopkins University Press.

Mennie ME, Gilfillan A, Compton ME, Liston WA, Brock DJ. (1993). "Prenatal cystic fibrosis carrier screening: factors in a woman's decision to decline testing." *Prenatal Diagnosis* 13: 807–14.

Mass, M., & AI-Krenawi, A. (1994). "When a man encounters a woman, Satan is also present: Clinical relationships in Bedouin society." *American Journal of Orthopsychiatry* 64: 357–67.

McAllister, M. (2001). "Grounded theory in genetic counseling research." *Journal of Genetic Counseling* 10(3): 233–51.

———. (1999). Predictive testing for hereditary nonpolyposis colorectal cancer: a theory of engagement. PhD thesis, University of Cambridge.

McCannell, Dean. (1976). "Staged Authenticity: Arrangements of Social Space in Tourist Settings," in his *The Tourist: A New Theory for the Leisure Class.* NY: Schoken.

Meir A, Barnea D. (1985). The Development of the Negev Bedouin educational system. Dept. of Geography. Beer-Sheva: Ben-Gurion University of the Negev.

Meir A. (1997). *As Nomadism Ends: The Israeli Bedouin of the Negev.* Boulder, CO: Westview Press.

Meir, Avinoam and Ben-David, Yosef (1995). "From latent surplus to changing norms: Fertility behavior of the Israeli Bedouin along the nomadism-sedentarism continuum," *Journal of Comparative Family Studies* 26(3): 389–409

Mendez, A. & Shymansky, J. (1984). "Verbal behaviors and patterns exhibited by physicians during genetic counselling sessions." *Patient Education and Counseling* 6(4): 165–68.

Mernissi, Fatima (1987). *Beyond the Veil: Male-Female Dynamics in Modem Muslim Society.* Bloomington: Indiana University Press.

Merton, R. (1957). *Social theory and social structure.* NY: Free Press.

Merz, B (1987). "Matchmaking scheme solves Tay-Sachs problem." *Journal of American Medical Association,* 258: 263–69.

Miadzybrodzka ZH, Hall ME, Mollison J, Templeton A, Russell IT, Dean JCS, Kelly KF, Marteau TM, Haites NE. (1995). "Antenatal screening for carriers of cystic fibrosis: randomised trial of stepwise versus couple screening." *British Medical Journal* 310: 353–57.

Michie S. Bron F, Bobrow M, Marteau TM. (1997a). "Nondirectiveness in Genetic counseling: an empirical study." *American Journal of Human Genetics* 60: 40–47.

Michie, S., French, D., Allanson, A. Bobrow, M. & Marteau, T. (1997b). "Information recall in genetic counseling: A pilot study of its assessment." *Patient Education and Counseling* 32: 93–100.

Michie, S. McDonald V., T. Marteau (1996). "Understanding response to predictive genetic testing: A grounded theory approach." *Psychological Health* 11: 455–70.

Middleton, A. J. Hewison & R. Nueller (2001). "Prenatal Diagnosis for deafness—what is the potential demand?" *Journal of genetic counseling* 10(2): 121–32.

Mishler E. (1984). *The discourse of medicine: The dialectics of medical interviews.* Norwood, NJ: Ablex.

Mitchell J, Capua A, Clow C, Scriver C. (1996) "Twenty-year outcome analysis of genetic screening programs for Tay-Sachs and [beta]-thalassemia disease carriers in high schools." *American Journal of Human Genetics* 59: 793–98.

Mittman, I. W. Crombleholme, J. Green & M. Golbus (1998). "Reproductive Genetic Counseling to Asian-Pacific and Latin American Immigrants." *Journal of Genetic Counseling* 7(1): 49–70.

Modell B, Harris R, Lane B, Khan M, Darlison M, Petrou M, Old J, Layton M, Varnavides L. (2000). "Informed choice in genetic screening for thalassaemia during pregnancy: audit from a national confidential inquiry." *British Medical Journal* 320: 337–41.

Modell, B. & V. Berdoukas (1984). *The Clinical Approach to Thalassemia.* London: Grune & Stratton.

Modell, B. & A. Kuliev (1991). "Services for thalassemia as a model for cost benefit analysis of genetic services." *Journal of Inherited Metabolic Diseases* 14: 640–51.

Nance, W. (1971). "Genetic Counseling for the Hearing Impaired." *Audiology* 10: 222–33.

————. (1977). "Genetic Counseling for the Hearing Impaired: An unmet need." In Bess, H (ed.), *Childhood Deafness: Causation, Assessment and Management.* NY: Grune and Stratton, pp. 211–16.

National Institutes of Health (United States) [NIH]—Working Group on Ethical, Legal, and Social Implications of the Human Genome Research [ELSI] Task Force on genetic testing (Neil A. Holtzman, chair). (1997). *Promoting Safe and Effective Genetic Testing in the United States: Principles and Recommendations.*

National Academy of Sciences and National Research Council. (1975). Genetic Screening: Programmes, Principles and Research. Washington: National Academy of Sciences.

National Society of Genetic counselors (1997). *What is Genetic Counseling?* Wallingford, PA.

Navarro, V. (1986). *Crisis, Health and Medicine: A Social Critique.* London: Tavistock.

Nelkin, D. & M. Lindee (1995). *The DNA Mystique: The Gene as a Cultural Icon.* NY: Freeman & Company.

Newman, I., & C. Benz. (1998). *Qualitative-Quantitative Research Methodology.* Carbonadale, IL: Southern Illinois University Press.

Nichter, M. (1999). "Project Community Diagnosis: Participatory research as a first step toward community involvement in primary health care." Pp. 300–27 in R. Hahn (ed.), *Anthropology in Public Health.* NY: Oxford University Press.

Nuffield Council on Bioethics (1993). *Genetic Screening: Ethical Issues.* London: Nuffield Council on Bioethics.

Omenn, G. (2000). "Public Health Genetics: An emerging interdisciplinary field for the post-genomic era," *Annual Review of Public Health* 21: 1–13.

Omran, Abd-el Rahim (1993). *Family Planning in the Legacy of Islam.* London: Routledge.

Padden, C. & T. Humphries. (1988). *Deaf in America—Voices from a Culture.* Cambridge, MA: Harvard University Press.

Panter-Brick C. (1991). "Parental responses to consanguinity and genetic disease in Saudi-Arabia." *Social Science & Medicine* 33: 1295–302.

Parens E, Asch A (Eds). (2000). *Prenatal Testing and Disability Rights.* Washington, DC: Georgetown University Press.

Pilnick, A. (2002). "'There are no rights and wrongs in these situations': identifying interactional difficulties in genetic counseling." *Sociology of Health & Illness* 24(1): 66–88.

Pilnick, A. & Dingwall, R. (2001). "Research directions in genetic counselling. A review of the literature." *Patient Education and Counseling* 44: 95–105.

Post, S., J. Botkin & P. Whitehouse (1992). "Selective abortion for familial Alzheimer Disease?" *Obstetrics and Gynecology* 79: 794–98.

President's Commission for the Study of Ethical Problems in Medicine and Biomedical and Behavioral Research, Screening and Counseling For Genetic Conditions: The Ethical, Social And Legal Implications Of Genetic Screening, Counseling, And Education Programs 18 (1983). Washington, D.C.

Rapp, Rayna (1998). "Refusing prenatal diagnosis: The meanings of bioscience in a multicultural world." *Science, Technology & Human Values* 23,1: 45–70.

———. (1999). *Testing Women, Testing the Fetus: The Social Impact of Amniocentesis in America.* New York: Routledge.

Raz, A. (1999). "Glocalization and Symbolic Interactionism," *Studies in Symbolic Interaction* 22: 3–16.

———. (2003). "Status disclosure: Genetic counseling as an arena for negotiation," *Studies in Symbolic Interaction*, 26: 41–61.

———. (2004). "Important to test, important to support: Attitudes towards disability rights and prenatal diagnosis among leaders of support groups for genetic disorders in Israel," forthcoming in *Social Science and Medicine.*

Resta, R. (1997). "Eugenics and Nondirectiveness in Genetic Counseling," *Journal of Genetic Counseling* 6: 255–58.

Rispler-Chaim, V. (1999). "The right not to be born: Abortion of the disadvantaged fetus in contemporary fatwas." *The Muslim World*, 89(2): 130–43.

Rogers, T. (1999). "The Islamic ethics of abortion in the traditional Islamic sources." *The Muslim World* 89(2): 122–29.

Rothman, Barbara (1986). *Tentative Pregnancy: Prenatal Diagnosis and the Future of Motherhood.* NY: Norton.

Sacks, Oliver (1989). *Seeing Voices: A Journey into the world of the deaf.* Berkeley: University of California Press.

———. (1997). *The Island of the Colorblind.* NY: Knopf.

Sagi, Mihal. (1998). "Genetic Screening in Israel," *Science in Context* 11(3–4): 419–31.

Scott DA, Kraft ML, Carmi R, Ramesh A, Elbedour K, Yairi Y, Srikumari CR, Rosengren SS, Markham AF, Mueller RF, Lench NJ, Van Camp G, Smith R JH, Sheffield VC. (1998). "Identification of mutations in the Connexin 26 gene that causes autosomal recessive nonsyndromic hearing loss." *Human Mutation* 11: 387–94.

Shakespeare, T. (1995). "Disabled people and the new genetics." *Genethics News* 5: 8–11.

Shamir, Ronen (1996). "Suspending in space: Bedouins under the law of Israel." *Law & Society Review* 30(2): 231–57.

Sharp, Richard & Morris Foster (2000). "Involving study populations in the review of genetic research." *The Journal of Law, Medicine & Ethics*, 28(1): 41–51.

Sher, Carron, Orly Romano-Zelekha, Manfred S. Green & Tamy Shohat (2003). "Factors affecting performance of prenatal genetic testing by Israeli Jewish women," *American Journal of Medical Genetics* 120A, 3: 418–22.

Shiloh, S. et al. (1995). "Premarital genetic counseling to consanguineous couples." *Social Sciences and Medicine*, 41(9): 1301–10.

Shohat, M., et al. (2003). "Prenatal diagnosis of Down syndrome: Ten year experience in the Israeli population" *American Journal of Medical Genetics* 122A(3): 215–22

Shuval, J. & O. Anson (2000). *Social Structure and Health in Israel.* Magnes Press, Jerusalem: The Hebrew University (in Hebrew).

Simpson, Bob (2000). "Imagined Genetic Communities." *Anthropology Today* 16(3): 3–8.

Sorensen, J., Kavanagh, C. & Mucatel, M. (1981). "Client learning of risk and diagnosis in genetic counseling." *Birth Defects* 17(11): 2115–228.

Stamatoyannopoulos G. (1974). "Problems of screening and counselling in the hemoglobinopathies." In: Motulsky AG, Lenz W, eds. *Birth defects*, Amsterdam, Excerpta Medica.

Stimson G. and Webb B. (1975). *Going to see the doctor: The consultation process in general practice.* London: Routledge Paul.

Strauss, Anselm. (1978). *Negotiations: Varieties, Contexts, Processes, and Social Order.* San Francisco: Jossey-Bass.

————. (1993). *Continual Permutations of Action.* New York: Aldine de Gruyter.

————. (1997). *Mirrors and Masks.* 2nd ed. New Brunswick, NJ: Transaction.

Strauss, Anselm, Shizuko Fagerhaugh, Barbara Suczek, and Carolyn Wiener,. (1997). *Social Organization of Medical Work.* New Brunswick, NJ: Transaction.

Strike, K. (2000). "Liberalism, communitarianism and the space between," *Journal of Moral Education* 29(2): 133–47.

Sue, D. & D. Sue. (1990). *Counseling the culturally different: Theory and practice.* NY: J. Wiley.

Sutton, A. (1990). *Prenatal Diagnosis: Confronting the Ethical Issues.* London: The Linacre Press.

Tan Alora, A & JM Lumitao (Eds.) (2001). *Beyond a western bioethics: Voices from the developing world.* Washington, DC: Georgetown UP.

Waitzkin, H. (1983). *The Second Sickness: The Contradictions of Capitalist Health care.* NY: Free Press.

———. (1991). *The Politics of Medical Encounters.* New Haven: Yale University Press.

Wallerstein, I. (1974). *The Modern World System.* NY: Academic Press.

Wang, V. & F. Marsh (1992). "Ethical principles and cultural integrity in health care delivery: Asian ethnocultural perspectives in genetic services." *Journal of Genetic Counseling* 1: 81–92.

Watson, B. (1999). "Liberal communitarianism as political theory," *Perspectives on Political Science* 28(4): 211–17.

Watson, M., Lloyd S., Eeles R., Ponder B., Easton D., Seal, S., Averill D., Daly P., Ormiston W., Murday V. (1996). "Psychosocial impact of testing (by linkage) for the BRCA1 breast cancer gene: An investigation of two families in the research setting." *Psychooncology* 5: 233–39.

Watson, M. Murday V., Lloyd S., Ponder B., Averill D., Eeles R. (1995). "Genetic testing in breast/ovarian cancer families." *Lancet* 346: 583.

Webster, A. (1984). *Introduction to the Sociology of Development.* London: Macmillan.

Weil, J. (2001). "Multicultural education and genetic counseling." *Clinical Genetics,* 59: 143–49.

Weil, J. and I. Mittman. (1993). "A teaching framework for cross-cultural genetic counseling." *Journal of Genetic Counseling* 2(3): 159–69.

Weiss, Meira (2002). *The Chosen Body: The Politics of the Body in Israeli Society.* Stanford: Stanford University Press.

Weitzman D, Shoham-Vardi I, ElBedour, K. Belmaker I, Siton Y. Carmi R. (2000). "Factors affecting utilization of prenatal testing for fetal abnormalities in a traditional society." *Community Genetics* 3(2): 45–92.

Wertz, D. (1998). "Eugenics is alive and well: A survey of genetic professionals around the world," *Science in Context* 3–4: 493–510.

Wertz, D. & J. Fletcher (1989). *Ethics and Human Genetics: A Cross-Cultural Perspective.* Heidelberg: Springer-Verlag.

Wiener, C. (2000). "Applying the Straussian Framework of Action, Negotiation, and Social Arenas to a Study of Accountability in Hospitals," *Sociological Perspectives* 43(4): S59.

WHO (2002). Genomics and World Health: Report of the Advisory Committee on Health Research. World Health Organization: Geneva.

WHO (1997). Community control of genetic and congenital disorders. EMRO Technical Publications Series, 24.

WHO (1985). "Community approaches to the control of hereditary diseases," unpublished WHO document HMG/AG/85.10. Hereditary Diseases Program, Geneva.

Wolff, G. & C. Jung (1995). "Nondirectiveness and genetic counseling." *Journal of Genetic Counseling* 4: 3–25.

Van Dijck, J. (1998). *Imagenation: Popular Images of Genetics.* NY: NY University Press.

Vital, David (1975). *The Origins of Zionism.* Oxford: Oxford University Press.

Young, L. (1992). "Sexual abuse and the problem of embodiment." *Child Abuse and Neglect* 16(1): 89–111.

Zeesman S., et al. (1984). "A private view of heterozygosity: Eight-year follow-up study on carriers of the Tay-Sachs gene detected by highschool screening in Montreal." *American journal of medical genetics*, 18: 769–78.

Zlotogora J, Leventhal A. (2000). "Screening for genetic disorders among Jews: How should the Tay-Sachs screening program be continued?" *Isr Med Assoc* J 2: 665–67.

Zola, I. (1972). "Medicine as an institution of social control." *Sociological Review* 20, 487–504.